Obstetrics and Gynaecology in General Practice:
the primary care handbook and aide memoire,
second edition

Obstetrics and Gynaecology in General Practice:
the primary care handbook and aide memoire,
second edition

Chris Barclay MB ChB MRCOG MFFP

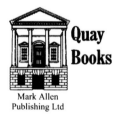

Quay Books

Mark Allen
Publishing Ltd

Quay Books Division of Mark Allen Publishing Limited
Jesse's Farm, Snow Hill, Dinton
Salisbury, Wiltshire SP3 5HN

British Library Cataloguing-in-Publication Data
A catalogue record is available for this book

ISBN 1 85642 164 3

Printed in the UK by Polestar Wheatons Limited, Exeter, Devon, UK

contents

Chapter 4 Preconceptual care 121

Chapter 5 Infertility 128

Chapter 6 Pregnancy and the puerperium(1) consequential conditions 136

Chapter 7 Pregnancy and the puerperium (2) coincidental conditions 173

Chapter 8 Breast disorders   193

Breast disorders in non-pregnant women   194

Breast disorders in pregnancy and the puerperium   200

Index   205

acknowledgements

I would like to thank sincerely several people who have encouraged or assisted in the production of this book. Firstly, thanks and blame in equal measure to my old school friend Steve Bazire (Buz) who deviously sowed the seed and patiently waited a week for me to come up with the idea.

Thanks especially to my long suffering partners Gay Forster, Ginny Bennett, Rachel Yates and Adrian Smith who, despite the upheaval and inconvenience, graciously allowed me time off to study. Thanks too to Trish' Broadbent who filled my shoes so professionally during my leave and who has since joined our partnership. More especial thanks for advice and comment on the text to Mr Peter Stewart, Mr TC Li, Mr Malcolm Reed, Dr Anton Shaw and Steve Bazire. Thanks also to Sue Whitaker and Sarah Copley for their support and encouragement.

Many thanks to Valery Marston and her staff at Quay Books for their patience, tolerance and skill in drawing a book out of the manuscript. My children Thomas, Hope and Miriam also request acknowledgement. And finally, thanks to my wife Beverley who has patiently tolerated my protracted literary gestation; a process which is as nothing (she tells me) compared with the real thing.

foreword

Although there have been notable developments since the first edition this book's key words remain, 'practising' and 'primary care'. This is a book for GPs by a GP. Women's health in today's general practice has surprisingly little in common with hospital based obstetrics and gynaecology. It is GPs who deal with most cases of menorrhagia and PMS, for example. Indeed, it is GPs who provide almost all the nation's family planning and menopausal services. I hope that this book will help GPs regain a degree of ownership of these services as it is they who are, in reality, the lead professionals in this rewarding area of healthcare.

This book is an aide memoire. Not something for the library but rather something to keep next to MIMS and the BNF in your consulting room. It may well be useful to those working on formularies and guidelines in their own practices and within primary care groups. It may also be of use to those working towards their DRCOG, DFFP and MRCGP examinations. But it is, above all, a pragmatic manual for general practitioners .

While trying to keep the data presented here evidence-based, I am sure some of my personal anecdotage will have crept in occasionally and for that I beg forgiveness. I would ask you to help me by offering correction and/or comment on the text. Your correspondence should be directed to Quay Books.

Chris Barclay
December, 1999

how to use this book

The primary remit of this book is to be a rapid reference and aide memoire during consultation with women. Each chapter is therefore organised in a way that seems appropriate for the subject. For those of you who wish to refer to it during patient contact, it is recommended that you familiarise yourself in advance with the content and layout of each of the chapters. This is a book for the consulting room, not the practice library.

1. **Gynaecological conditions** Data on conditions important to primary care professionals are presented alphabetically. They have been selected because they are either common or important in the primary care setting. Data on management at the secondary/tertiary care level is not discussed.

2. **The change** This chapter looks at the climacteric and was the most thorny to write. Specific data is listed under the principal therapeutic agent headings. Numerous tables display data that will be of use during consultation. Some study of the issues on prophylactic use of HRT is recommended as professional opinions inevitably remain subjective even after weighing the evidence. New data on HRT and breast cancer is included. The recently introduced SERMs are discussed. Heretics are no longer burned.

3. **Contraception** All primary care contraceptive options are presented in this chapter. Detailed answers to commonly posed questions are listed in an A–Z fashion under each method. Data on the full range of contraceptive options available in British primary care can be located using the Chapter Contents and in the numerous Tables and Information Boxes. Recent additions to the text have been made regarding the Persona, Gynefix IUD and the new data on progestogen-only contraception.

4. **Preconceptual preparation** like emergency contraception, should not just be available, it must be prospectively offered. Well woman check-ups, attendance for contraception and even postnatal visits and child immunisation clinics provide excellent opportunities for advertising your preconceptual wares when women may be most receptive. Data is presented in an A–Z fashion under three headings (aims, clinical questions, check-lists).

5. **Fertility questions** are presented in a pragmatic way. I envisage that the interested professional would be able to 'workup' couples and in appropriate cases perhaps even administer and supervise clomiphene oral ovulation induction therapy.

6. **Pregnancy and the puerperium (1) consequential conditions** Data for the primary care professional on common or important antenatal problem areas are listed alphabetically. The management of labour and delivery is not considered a basic primary care topic (although many primary care professionals will be involved in delivering this community-based secondary care service) and it is therefore beyond the scope of this chapter. With childbirth arrangements changing it may become a feature of subsequent editions.

7. **Pregnancy and the puerperium (2) coincidental conditions** This chapter lists a variety of conditions and therapies that are either important or encountered with some frequency in women of childbearing age. I have tried to avoid overlap with the previous chapter by concentrating here on conditions and therapies incidental to pregnancy. In appropriate instances, data is presented in tabular form only.

8. **Breast disease** Data in this chapter is collected under two headings (disorders in pregnancy and the puerperium and those unrelated to pregnancy), and aims to cover most primary care presentations of breast disorder. Breast cancer, although of paramount importance, is only briefly discussed as its diagnosis is generally made in the secondary care setting.

1
gynaecology

Data on conditions important to primary care professionals are presented alphabetically. They have been selected because they are either common or important in the primary care setting. Data on management at the secondary/tertiary care level is not discussed.

Chapter contents

acne vulgaris

amenorrhoea

bacterial vaginosis

bartholins gland disease

cancer

candidiasis

cervical polyp

cervicitis

DES exposure

dysmenorrhoea

dyspareunia

ectopic pregnancy

endometriosis

fibroids

hirsutism

infection

intraepithelial neoplasia

labial adhesion

menstrual disturbance

miscarriage (abortion)

ovarian cyst

ovulation pain

pelvic inflammatory disease

pelvic pain syndrome

polycystic ovary syndrome

premenstrual syndrome

prolactinoma

prolapse

psychosexual problems

screening in gynaecology

toxic shock syndrome

trophoblastic disease

urinary incontinence

vaginal discharge

vulval disorder

Tables

Acne vulgaris

Although a dermatological condition acne vulgaris has a place in an aide memoire on gynaecology (see also 'Skin conditions coinciding with pregnancy', *Chapter 6*).

- **abnormal androgen production** can produce acne as well as hirsutism. In severe cases defeminisation and masculinisation can occur too. Consider adrenal hyperplasia and adrenal and ovarian androgen secreting tumours

- **combined oral contraceptive pill** generally leads to an improvement in the skin of acne sufferers. Occasionally acne develops in pill users. In that instance, a less androgenic pill (see *Chapter 3*) or a third generation pill can be tried

- **contraceptive failure** can result from initial treatment of acne with tetracyclines and erythromycins. It is, however, generally assumed that long term low dose use of these antibiotics is safe in combination with the pill. The mechanism for failure in the first two or three weeks of treatment is bowel flora disturbance, affecting enterohepatic oestrogen circulation before a steady state resumes. Changing antibiotics can produce a further disturbance in bowel flora

- **Dianette** is a contraceptive pill combining ethinyloestradiol 35mcg and cyproterone acetate 2mg. Cyproterone is an anti-androgen and produces a response similar to that of oral antibiotics. It reduces sebum production and also has a beneficial effect in women with hirsutism. The dose of cyproterone is small (a usual dose used in carcinoma of the prostate for example is 200 mg/day). Dianette is contraindicated in pregnancy and in women breast feeding. It can cause liver anomalies and has the usual cautions and contraindications associated with the combined pill. Treatment is usually stopped when a good response is seen. Repeat courses can be given

- **drug induced acne** is seen with the use of androgenic progestogens especially at the higher doses found in Depo-Provera and Noristerat. It can follow use of Norplant and, occasionally, Mirena as well as the combined and progestogen only pills. Acne can follow steroid therapy and can be mimicked by contact with certain chemicals

- **teratogenesis** can occur with drugs used in the treatment of acne vulgaris. Oxytetracycline and related tetracyclines damage bones and teeth. Dianette is anti-androgenic and could cause fetal anomaly. Vitamin A derivatives, especially isotretinoin (Roaccutane) must not be given in pregnancy. In addition, women should have effective contraception at least one month before and for one month after therapy. Topical isotretinoin and tretinoin are also contraindicated in pregnancy

Amenorrhoea

May be a primary or secondary phenomenon.

Primary amenorrhoea arbitrarily defined as absence of menarche by around the age of 16 years. Investigation should be considered earlier if by 14 years there are no signs of secondary sexual development either. The presence or absence of secondary sexual characteristics is crucial. Causes to be considered include:

- **physiological:** no disease, end of normal range
- **endocrine disorder (non- virilising):** thyroid dysfunction
- **endocrine disorder (virilising):** adrenal or ovarian tumour, congenital adrenal hyperplasia
- **genetic anomaly**: Turner's syndrome, testicular feminisation (now known as androgen insensitivity syndrome), hypothalamic (Kallman's syndrome), intersex
- **genital tract anomaly**: absence of uterus or ovaries, congenital obstruction to passage of menses by stenosis, atresia or imperforate hymen

investigation

Initially involves personal and family history followed by assessment of physical and secondary sexual development including, if permitted by the patient, external genital examination. Look for stigmata of pathological causes, eg. wide spaced nipples and neck webbing of Turner's syndrome. Early referral for secondary opinion to avoid distressing duplication of examination and blood tests is acceptable.

treatment

Depends entirely on the outcome of investigations and is a secondary or even tertiary management case.

Secondary amenorrhoea arbitrarily defined as cessation of menstruation for more than six months.

- **physiological**: pregnancy, lactation and the menopause
- **endocrine anomaly**: in addition to ovarian failure and PCOS it is essential to exclude a pituitary adenoma by measuring serum prolactin. If this is marginally raised repeat the test. If it is markedly raised or if there are headaches or visual disturbance a secondary opinion is mandatory. Hypothyroidism is often quoted, but is a rare cause
- **hypothalamic disorder**: classically in anorexia nervosa and in athletes with minimal body fat
- **polycystic ovary syndrome**: see section below
- **post-pill amenorrhoea** is probably a modern myth. It is generally preceded by pre-pill menstrual disturbance
- **premature ovarian failure** can occur from the late teens onwards. It may be a familial trait or it may be the consequence of genetic abnormality eg. 47 XXX karyotype
- **rarities**: resistant ovary syndrome where the ovary appears to hibernate and the menopause is mimicked. Sheehan's syndrome of hypopituitarism following massive haemorrhage, and Asherman's syndrome usually following vigorous uterine curettage removing all the endometrial tissue and often producing

intrauterine synechiae (comparable with successful endometrial ablation)

- **virilising condition**: if defeminisation has occurred or virilisation is developing, adrenal hyperplasia and adrenal and ovarian tumour need urgently excluding. Secondary referral urgent

investigation

After full external examination and exclusion of pregnancy (almost always worth doing) check serum gonadotrophins and prolactin. More intensive endocrine workup includes SHBG, androstendione, oestradiol and testosterone. Karyotype if indicated. Refer for secondary opinion if fertility questions are important or if significant pathology suspected. If premature menopause is the cause (climacteric symptoms, low oestradiol, grossly raised FSH) consider HRT and osteoporosis workup.

treatment

- aim to reassure women with no pathology
- investigate any pathology appropriately
- investigate further if future pregnancy may be desired
- investigate urgently if defeminisation has occurred
- refer urgently if virilisation is present

Bacterial vaginosis

Formerly known as haemophillus vaginalis, and gardnerella vaginitis. Bacterial vaginosis (BV) is a condition or state of having an abnormal vaginal bacterial flora. A variety of anaerobes can be implicated. It is common, one study found that 12% of affluent antenatal patients and 28% of women requesting termination of pregnancy tested positive. It is frequently asymptomatic. Should anything be done for women in whom it is identified?

Diagnostic features

- **vaginal pH** >4.5 The normally strongly acidic vaginal pH rises as protective lactobacilli are displaced. Do not apply 10% KOH directly to the vaginal skin as it will cause a chemical burn
- **grey homogenous vaginal discharge** may be complained of or noted on examination
- **presence of 'clue cells'** on wet mount preparations. The clue was finding a stippling change over the surface membrane of vaginal epithelial cells caused by adherent bacteria
- **amine test** is positive in BV. The amines are volatile fishy smelling odours which are released if a drop of 10% potassium hydroxide is applied to a smear of the vaginal discharge on a glass slide. Seminal fluid being alkaline can also cause an embarrassing fishy odour to develop during sexual intercourse

Clinical features

- **asymptomatic BV,** in the absence of an IUD, and in the absence of pregnancy or a desire to become pregnant or other indication, should probably be ignored. Treating such women is in fact treating the laboratory result, not the patient
- **ineffective treatments** include erythromycin, tetracycline, povidone-iodine, acetic acid, dienoestrol and intravaginal lactobacillus
- **IUD contraception:** it is good practice to take a bacteriological swab prior to IUD insertion. Whether asymptomatic BV should be treated in this situation is not known
- **male sexual partners** do not require concurrent treatment. It is ineffective
- **pregnancy**: it is thought that BV can cause late miscarriage and preterm labour. Trials are currently under way assessing the benefit (and detriments) of BV eradication therapy in pregnancy. For the time being, treatment of asymptomatic women can not be advised in pregnancy. If it is proposed to treat symptomatic infection (discharge, odour) it should be done in conjunction with an obstetrician
- **pre-pregnancy** identification of BV and treatment has not been advocated in published data, but if it was discovered it would be difficult to withhold treatment knowing that BV can cause adverse pregnancy outcome
- **post abortal sepsis** is linked with BV. Many gynaecologists screen for BV and other opportunistic and pathogenic infections prior to termination of pregnancy
- **vaginal discharge** in the presence of BV should be treated
- **vaginal odour** in the presence of BV should be treated

Table 1.1: Treatments available for bacterial vaginosis

Metronidazole oral treatment, either 2 g as a stat dose or 400 mg tds for one week (one regime mentioned 500 mg bd for 5 or 7 days). Metronidazole is available as 200 mg, 400 mg tabs, and as a suspension 200 mg/5 ml. Topical treatment: metronidazole pessaries, 1g pv nocte for two days *Caution*: Disulfuram (antabuse) reaction with alcohol, pregnancy and breast feeding, liver disease. *Interactions*: alcohol and disulfuram enhances anticoagulant effect of nicoumalone and warfarin, inhibits metabolism of phenytoin and fluorouracil, increases risk of lithium toxicity, phenobarbitone and cimetidine enhances effects of metronidazole
Metronidazole vaginal gel; 40 g of 0.75% gel with 5 applicators. One applicatorful to be inserted intravaginally each night for five consecutive nights. Not to be used in first trimester of pregnancy. May interact with lithium and alcohol. May cause GI upset and vaginal irritation. No data on effect on latex, eg. in condoms and contraceptive diaphragms
Tinidazole oral treatment, 500 mg bd for one week or 2 g stat dose. Tinidazole is available as film-coated tabs 500mg. *Cautions* same as metronidazole
Clindamycin topical treatment: vaginal gel 2%, 5 g pv daily for one week. Available as 40 g pack with 7 applicators. The gel can damage latex in condoms, diaphragms and caps. Post treatment candidiasis is reported. Be alert to remote risk of pseudomembranous colitis Oral treatment: clindamycin capsules 300 mg bd for seven days.

References

Review paper. MacDermot RIJ (1995) *Br J Obstet Gynaecol* **102**: 92–4

RSM (1993) The diagnosis and management of bacterial vaginosis. *Proceedings of a round table discussion*, No 30

Bartholin's gland disease

Most diagnoses of Bartholin's gland cyst or abscess are incorrect. Sebaceous cysts are common in the hair bearing areas of the vulva. The Bartholin's glands are in fact situated postero-laterally just deep to the skin in the vestibule, not the vulva (at the 4 and 8 o'clock positions). Bartholin's cysts therefore bulge from the side of the perineum into the lower vagina and vestibule. There are numerous other smaller and un-named mucous glands in the vestibule that can produce cystic swellings.

The anatomical distinctions are of some consequence as sebaceous cysts are usually quite trivial and of little significance. Bartholin's gland cysts and abscess, on the other hand, may be markers for sexually transmitted disease and referral for a specialist genito-urinary consultation should be considered. Surgical treatment by a gynaecologist is often required too. Malignancy is exceedingly rare.

Cancer

Gynaecological malignancy is not uncommon. Treatments are almost exclusively the province of the specialist except for palliative and symptomatic treatment. The incidence of female genital tract cancers are shown in *Table 1.2*.

Table 1.2: Incidence of gynaecological cancers in women under 75 years of age

	New cancer registrations in 1983	Cancer deaths in 1985
cervix	1591 (1.6%)	3426 (4.6%)
uterus	781 (0.8%)	2967 (3.9%)
ovary	2788 (2.7%)	3547 (4.7%)

(*Womens Health Today*. Office of Health Economics, N Wells. 1987)

Bartholin's gland cancer

Tumours are an exceeding rarity.

- **incidence**: in a study from New York, this was slightly greater than one case per million woman years among postmenopausal women
- **presentation**: in the postmenopausal years with a mass or cyst bulging from the posterolateral aspect of the vestibule. Diagnosis is by biopsy

Cervical cancer

Most tumours are squamous although a few are adenocarcinomas. Invasive disease in the presence of an adequate smear history is rare. Diagnosis is often made by cone biopsy. Treatment depends on staging of the disease. Options are either surgical, including Wertheim's hysterectomy with lymph node dissection and/or radiotherapy which can be administered externally or internally:

- **incidence**: the second commonest of the gynaecological cancers. Most present in women 40–70 years
- **presentation**: microinvasive disease is asymptomatic. Abnormal vaginal bleeding (intermenstrual, post coital, during pregnancy or post menopausal) should always raise the question of malignancy. Cervical ulceration or mass requires urgent referral

Fallopian tube cancer

This is a rarity which is often only diagnosed at operation or occasionally on histological evidence. It mimics ovarian cancer clinically:

- **incidence**: exceedingly rare, 0.3% of female genital tract cancer
- **presentation**: usually mimics ovarian cyst or tumour. Peak incidence at 55 years, 50% are in nulliparous women

Ovarian cancer

Ninety percent are epithelial. The remainder include stromal and germ cell derived tumours. The ovary may be the host for secondary deposits from other primary cancers. A family history of ovarian cancer increases the lifetime risk significantly. See screening for ovarian cancer in section on 'screening in gynaecology' below:

- **incidence**: the commonest malignant female genital tract tumour
- **presentation**: sadly is frequently with secondary disease; ascites, pleural effusion, general debility. Occasionally an early stage tumour is detected fortuitously during examination for other reasons, eg. cervical smear testing

Uterine cancer

Most tumours are endometrial cancers although leiomyosarcomas arising from the myometrium or within fibroids do occur. The higher background oestrogen levels seen in obese postmenopausal women predispose them to endometrial cancer:

- **incidence**: ninth commonest female cancer (3%)
- **presentation**: classically with postmenopausal bleeding although endometrial cancer can occur in premenopausal women. Abnormal vaginal bleeding in women in their mid to late forties should prompt investigation for endometrial cancer. Three quarters of patients are over 50 years at presentation

Vaginal cancer

This is uncommon. Most are related to cervical disease and are squamous in origin. Clear cell carcinoma of the vagina is well known in young women exposed *in utero* to diethylstilboestrol (see below):

- **incidence**: squamous cancers occur mainly in the elderly. High association with CIN. Adenocarcinoma which may be related to DES exposure and presents at any age
- **presentation**: early cases often noted by colposcopists during attendance for investigation of cervical disease. Otherwise as pain, bleeding and vaginal discharge

Vulval cancer

Vulval cancer is strongly associated with cervical disease and exposure to HPV. Tumours in the skin of the vulva, perineum and perianal areas have similar aetiologies, presentations and courses. Lymphoma can present as a vulval tumour as can malignant melanoma. Women with chronic vulval skin disorders or symptoms should be screened regularly, see vulval disorder below:

- **incidence**: uncommon. Generally a tumour of older women, but may occur in women in their 20s
- **presentation**: as an abnormality in the skin of the vulva, vestibule, perineum or perianal skin. Association with ano-rectal cancer

Candidiasis

Synonymous with 'yeast' or 'thrush' infection, around 90% of vulvovaginal candida infection are due to the albicans species. The majority of the remainder are caused by C. glabrata (Torulopsis glabrata). Resistant and recurrent candidiasis is more likely to be due to C. glabrata. Repetitive exposure to topical preparations increases resistance.

Candida is a commensal organism that causes opportunistic infections. The commonest situations for this are antibiotic therapy, pregnancy and diabetes mellitus. However, in most instances, the question is not 'where did she get thrush from?' rather it is 'why has she become susceptible to thrush in the first place?' Isolated single attacks of genital tract infection with candida organisms are extremely common. Recurrent attacks of candidiasis are a considerable source of irritation and discomfort.

Clinical questions

- **antibiotic therapy**, especially using broad spectrum agents, depletes the natural vaginal flora allowing overgrowth of opportunists. It has to be said that women generally take antibiotics when they are ill and the illness itself may reduce resistance too. Use of narrower range antibiotics can reduce this problem
- **clothing choice** is a factor. The warmer and more humid the genital area becomes the more susceptible it is to fungal infection. The skin of the vulva is second only to the axilla in transpiration of moisture; it needs ventilation
- **diabetes mellitus** can lead to excessive glucose in secretions favouring the growth of candida
- **gastro-intestinal tract therapy** has been shown to be ineffective in preventing recurrent disease. Adding a daily helping of live yoghurt to the diet, which contains the bacterium *lacto-bacillus acidophilus*, is said to be of benefit
- **immunosuppression**, like diabetes, can allow fungal overgrowth in many

locations. HIV must be considered in recurrent vulvovaginal candidiasis

- **iron deficiency** is no longer considered a causative factor. The same applies to zinc deficiency
- **male partner treatment** has been shown to be ineffective, even though analysis shows that the same serotype of candida may be harboured in the male urethra
- **oral contraception** is no longer considered a causative factor with the low dose pill, although it is often blamed. There is dispute about a causative role for 50mcg formulations
- **pregnancy** is associated with an increase in vaginal secretions and a lessening of immunological resistance making candida more frequent. Oral azole antifungals are contraindicated in pregnancy (itraconazole and fluconazole). Nystatin may be used although data is lacking. Systemic absorption of oral nystatin is said to be negligible. Topical azoles are the mainstay of treatment which may have to be given at a higher dose and for longer than usual

- **recurrent candidiasis** may be due to incorrect diagnosis, resistant albicans forms or presence of glabrata forms which are not infrequently resistant to the azoles. Diabetes and HIV should be considered. Submitting microbiological specimens for strain typing and sensitivities and discussion with the local microbiology laboratory is advisable. In persistent cases referral for a GUMed opinion is also an option. Intermittent prophylactic treatments with antifungals have been suggested. Regular application of topical antifungals or oral azole once or twice a month, until three to six months without relapse has ensued, is recommended
- **sexual transmission** is not thought to occur, rather thrush is associated with sexual activity causing trauma and minor abrasions. Adequate vaginal lubrication either physiologically or applied externally can help

---

Principles of drug treatment

The various *BNF* listed antifungal preparations are listed in *Tables 1.3–1.5*. Creams for intravaginal application come with applicators.

azole antifungals (topicals) See *Table 1.3*

These are the mainstay of therapy. Some preparations are available over the counter:

- **clotrimazole** creams are available in three strengths. The 10% preparation is for single dose intravaginal therapy and comes with an applicator. The 2% cream is similar but should be used BD for three days or nocte for six. 1% cream is for external use. The 500 mg pessary is a stat dose. The 100 mg vaginal tablets can be given as 2 nocte for three nights or 1 nocte for six nights
- **econazole** comes in similar formulations with a 150 mg stat dose form as well as three night regimes. 1% cream is available in topical or intravaginal formulations (*Table 1.3*)
- **fenticonazole** pessaries are soft and pliable and come in stat and three night courses
- **isoconazole** is presented in two 300 mg pessaries which should be inserted together as a stat nocte dose
- **ketoconazole** cream is for external use. The oral preparation can cause liver damage
- **miconazole** cream is available in intravaginal and topical formulations. Pessaries are for use on seven consecutive nights. Two stat dose intravaginal preparations are available; the ovule and the soft pessary (*Table 1.3*)

azole antifungals (oral) See *Table 1.3*

These are available in two formulations. Both are contraindicated in pregnancy and lactation. They may be marginally more effective than topical preparations and are less 'messy'. They are of course more costly:

- *fluconazole* is given as a single stat dose
- *itraconazole* is given as two doses of two capsules twelve hours apart

combination preparations

These come in two groups. The first are the same drug combinations in different vehicles (Canesten duopak, Ecostatin twinpack, Daktarin combipack). These are listed in *Table 1.3*. The second are antifungal combinations with other agents (*Table 1.5*). These additives include topical corticosteroids, antiseptics and antibacterials. The azoles are only available in combination with corticosteroids. Many are general dermatological preparations and some contain steroids of high potency. The antifungal/hydrocortisone preparations are the most useful choices in candidiasis of the vulva and vestibule.

Table 1.3: Single agent azole antifungals

Drug	Trade name	Presentation	Pack size	Latex damage	OTC
topical					
clotrimazole	Canesten	non-proprietary pessary 500 mg	1	ND	
		cream 1% (T)	20g; 50 g	?	√
		cream 10% (VC)	5g	?	
		vag tab 100 mg	3 or 6	ND	
		vag tab 200 mg	3	ND	√
		vag tab 500 mg	1*	ND	
		Canesten combi cream 1% tab 100 mg	6 plus 20 g	?	
	Masnoderm	cream 1%	20 g	+	√
econazole	Ecostatin	cream 1% (T)	15g, 30 g	+	√
		pessary 150 mg	1 or 3 *	+	
		twinpack pess 150 mg cream	3 plus 15 g 1% (T)	+	
	Gyno-Pevaryl	cream 1% (V)	15g; 30g	–	√
		CP pack 150 mg pessary 1% cream	1 plus 15 g	+	
		combipack 150 mg pessary 1% cream	3 plus 15 mg	+	
		pessary 150 mg	1 or 3 *	+	
	Pevaryl	cream 1% (T)	30 g	ND	√
fenticonazole	Lomexin	pessary 200 mg	3	+	
		pessary 600 mg	1	+	

Table 1.3: Single agent azole antifungals contin.

isoconazole	Travogyn	vag tab 300 mg	2	+	
ketoconazole	Nizoral	cream 2% (T)	30 g	ND	
		tabs 200 mg	ND	ND	
miconazole	Gyno-Daktarin	cream 2% (V)	78 g	+	
		pessary 100 mg	14	+	
		ovule 1.2 g	1	+	
		combipack pess and cream	14 plus 15 g (T)	+	
	Femeron	cream 2% (T)**	15g	+	√
		soft pessary 1.2 g	1	+	√
oral azoles					
itraconazole	Sporanox C/I	caps 100 mg	4		
fluconazole	Diflucan C/I	cap 150 mg	1		

Notes:

+	known to damage latex in condoms, caps and diaphragms
*	presented as a single dose formula with suffix '1' after drug name eg 'Canesten 1'
**	not available as NHS preparation
T	cream or gel for topical use
V	cream for vaginal use
S/P	special precaution
ND	no data
C/I	contraindicated
OTC	over the counter

Principal sources: *MIMS*, November 1999; *BNF* **38**, *September 1999*

polyene antifungals (nystatin) See *Table 1.4*

These are less often used now because they require a two week course to be effective and the topical creams should be applied between 2–4 times a day. The cream formulation stains underwear yellow. The oral tablets which are designed to clear the gastrointestinal reservoir of infection are ineffective prophylactically. Numerous combination preparations exist (*Table 1.5*) most of which are for general dermatological rather than vulvovaginal use.

non-pharmacological and other measures

The most important measures appear to be attention to clothing so that the vulval area can 'breath', avoidance of irritants, ensuring adequate lubrication during intercourse (endogenous or applied) and avoiding broad spectrum antibiotics. Treatment with minerals is of no help. Avoiding fermented and 'yeast' foods is suggested by some with little evidence of benefit. Artificial sweeteners which are not utilised in humans can provide a substrate for yeasts and have lead some to suggesting their avoidance. Adding live yoghurt with *lactobacillus acidophilus* is advised by some. Others advise instilling live yoghurt intravaginally to soothe symptoms and replenish acid producing flora. Aci-jel is available OTC and on prescription. It has a pH of 4 and is indicated in non-specific infections (one applicatorful BD to restore vaginal acidity).

Table 1.4: Single agent polyene antifungals

Drug	Trade name	Presentation	Pack size	Latex damage
polyenes				
nystatin	Nystan	vag cream 100 Ku/4 g (V)	60 g	+
		pessary 100 Ku	28	√

Notes:

+	known to damage latex in condoms, caps and diaphragms
T	cream or gel for topical use
V	cream for vaginal use

Table 1.5: Combination antifungals

Antifungal drug	Trade name	Combination drug	Presentation	Pack size	P
Azoles					
clotrimazole 1%	Canesten HC	hydrocortisone 1%	cream	30 g	1
	Lotriderm	betamethasone 0.05%	cream	15 g	3
econazole 1%	Econacort	hydrocortisone 1%	cream	30 g	1
	Pevaryl TC	triamcinolone 0.1%	cream	15 g	3
miconazole 2%	Daktacort	hydrocortisone 1%	cream and ointment	30 g	1
Polyenes					
nystatin 100Ku/g	Gregoderm	hydrocortisone 1% neomycin, polymyxin	ointment	15 g	1
	Nystaform-HC	hydrocortisone 0.5% chlorhexidene	cream and ointment	30 g	1
	Terra-Cortril Nystatin	hydrocortisone 1% oxytetracyclin	cream	30 g	1
	Timodene	hydrocortisone 0.5% benzalkonium dimethicone	cream	30 g	1
	Dermovate NN	clobetasol p 0.05% neomycin	cream and ointment	30 g	4
	Trimovate	clobetasone b 0.05% oxytetracycline	cream	30 g	2
	Nystadermal	triamcinolone 0.1%	cream	15 g	3
	Tri-Adcortyl	triamcinolone 0.1% gramicidin, neomycin	cream or ointment	30 g	3

Principal sources: *MIMS*, November 1999; *BNF* **38**, September 1999

Notes: all these preparations are for topical external use

P denotes steroid potency (1: mild; 2: moderate; 3: potent; 4: very potent)

Useful reading

British Society for Medical Mycology (1995) Management of genital candidiasis. Working group of the British Society for Medical Mycology. *Br Med J* **310**: 1241–4

White D (1995) Vaginal thrush; effective management. *The Practitioner* **239**: 612–6

Spinillo A *et al* (1995) Torulopsis glabrata vaginitis. *Obstet Gynecol* **85**: 993–8

Cervical polyp

Three varieties of polyp can present at the cervix:

Small inflammatory polyps

Most of these can be nipped off easily with silver nitrate cautery to control slight bleeding from the base. Tissue should always be submitted for histological analysis. A cytological smear should be taken unless a recent result is available. If in any doubt refer for secondary opinion.

Neoplastic polyps

True neoplastic polyps of cervix often arise from the lining of the endocervical canal. They are less granular and are not so easily removed in the primary care setting. Difficult to distinguish from uterine polyps. It is important that the polyp base is curetted as well and examined histologically along with the polyp itself. These polyps can bleed on removal and so should be referred on. Most will be benign.

Uterine polyps

Uterine polyps presenting via the cervical os especially endometrial and fibroid polyps. All should be referred on to a gynaecologist.

In all cases a contemporaneous cervical cytological report should be available or a cytological smear should be performed.

Cervicitis

Just as most vaginal discharges are physiological secretions rather than pathological emissions a red cervix is not necessarily an inflamed one. Genital tract infection must be sought with diligence but appending a pathological label may sometimes be inappropriate.

Cervical ectropion

This describes a cervix where the squamo-columnar junction is visible. The peripheral squamous skin surrounds the moist red glandular columnar epithelium. Ectropion is common in young women and in users of the combined oral contraceptive pill. If asymptomatic and in the face of a negative cytology report (and microbiology reports too if desired) it can be ignored. An excessive amount of vaginal secretion is sometimes attributed to ectropion and in this circumstance cryocautery or diathermy may be indicated if cytology is negative.

Nabothian follicles

Nabothian follicles occur under the transformation zone. This is the area of squamous epithelium that covers what was once columnar. This metaplastic change can occlude residual mucous gland ostia allowing mucous retention cysts to develop, ie. they are the consequence of metaplasia not infection.

True cervicitis

This produces a reddened inflamed cervix almost always associated with a mucoid or mucopurulent discharge. Chlamydia and gonococcal infections must be excluded and referral to a GU Medicine department is strongly recommended.

Diethylstilbestrol (DES) exposure

DES was used between 1940–1973 for a number of pregnancy associated conditions. The principal indications were in the treatment of threatened abortion and in the prevention of abortion in subsequent pregnancies. Around ten thousand women in England and Wales were given it in early pregnancy. There were numerous other indications (full review: Stillman RJ (1982) *Am J Obstet Gynecol* **142**: 905–21. See also *DTB* (1991) **29**: 49–50.

In the early 1950s, randomised trials failed to demonstrate any benefits in those treated. In the 1970s an epidemic of clear cell vaginal adenocarcinomas was noted and DES was found to be the cause. Its use was banned in the US in 1973. Subsequent analysis of old data has shown that the use of DES actually increased pregnancy complications; in other words, it was a therapy with risk but no benefit.

Clinical implication today

women exposed in utero

- *vaginal adenosis* describes the presence of columnar glandular epithelium over the cervix and onto the vaginal skin. It is extremely common in *in utero* DES exposed women (two thirds have it). It is similar to, but much more extensive than, the physiological ectropion of the cervix. As in the physiological situation the vaginal adenosis will, given time, transform to squamous epithelium and does not of itself require invasive treatment. A large transformation zone, extending well on to the vagina will develop. Screening and review should be given by a colposcopist

- *vaginal cancer* although more common is still a rarity. It is of the clear cell variety and presents in adolescence. The risk appears to diminish after the teenage years. It affects 0.14–1.4/1000 DES exposed daughters. This is 100–1000 times the natural expected incidence

- *cervico-vaginal dysplasia* is increased. It may be due to the much larger size of the transformation zone. Hence the need for colposcopic follow up

- *Mullerian anomalies* ranging from collars and hoods over the cervix, cervical incompetence to uterine and fallopian structural anomalies occur

- *fertility* may be compromised by DES exposure. This can result from anatomical anomaly, menstrual disturbance, poor cervical mucus and an increase in spontaneous abortion. Preterm delivery, low birth weight, toxaemia, malpresentation, ante-partum haemorrhage and perinatal mortality statistics are worse among DES exposed daughters

- **ectopic gestation** is more common among women exposed to DES
- **breast disease incidence** could be affected because of its hormone dependent status. Careful follow up is advised

women directly exposed in pregnancy

- **Women directly exposed in pregnancy** may have a higher incidence of breast cancer

men exposed in utero

- **anatomical anomaly** including microphallus, urethral stenosis, hypospadias, testicular anomalies, cryptorchidism and anomalies of the prostatic utricle
- **fertility** is decreased in exposed men by decreasing sperm quantity and quality

Useful address

For women offering or seeking information on DES:

Register of DES affected women in the UK, c/o Michelle Cowan MSc, 8 Groveside Close, London W3 0DX

Dysmenorrhoea

Painful periods can be classified into primary or spasmodic dysmenorrhoea and secondary or congestive dysmenorrhoea.

Primary dysmenorrhoea

This is a feature of ovulatory cycles. It is spasmodic and cramping and is due to uterine contractions. Simple analgesics are often sufficient. NSAIDs are particularly useful as they combine analgesia with a direct action on the cyclo-oxygenase system, inhibiting the formation of the pain causing prostaglandin F2α. Commonly used NSAIDs (mefenamic acid, ibuprofen, naproxen, diclofenac) are effective. They should be taken as short courses. Their efficacy is increased if they are commenced before the onset of menstruation, but this should only be advised where there is no risk of pregnancy. Aspirin has analgesic effects, but does not inhibit Pg F2α production.

Another useful alternative is the combined oral contraceptive pill. One small study found transdermal GTN (given as one quarter of a 10mg GTN patch applied daily) reduced period pain and interference with daily activities. Patch pieces were applied abdominally when pain began and applied daily until pain subsided (Pittrof R *et al*, 1996).

Secondary dysmenorrhoea

This is a pathological symptom and is characterised by constant dull pains which begin before the onset of menstruation. It is the result of inflammation, not colic. Treatment depends on the cause of the pain. Causes include:

- adenomyosis
- endometriosis
- pelvic venous congestion

- pelvic inflammatory disease
- psychological disorder.

Treatment is entirely dependent on aetiology. A low threshold for referral for a secondary care opinion is advisable. While awaiting an opinion baseline investigations can be started (FBC, MSU, bacteriology) and simple measures, as outlined under primary dysmenorrhoea, can be instituted. A high index of suspicion must be maintained in any woman with secondary dysmenorrhoea. The diagnoses of endometriosis and pelvic infection needs to be actively excluded. Endometriosis classically causes congestive secondary dysmenorrhoea which typically will have been present for many years before the diagnosis is made. Early referral is strongly advised to prevent progresson of the disease.

Reference

Pittrof R *et al* (1996) Crossover trial of glyceryl trinitrate patches for controlling pain in women with severe dysmenorrhoea. *Br Med J* **312**: 884

Dyspareunia

Dyspareunia or pain with intercourse is classified as superficial or deep depending on where the discomfort is felt.

Superficial dyspareunia

This is felt either on the vulva or vestibule and frequently precludes vaginal penetration:

- *hymenal remnants* are an occasional cause. Bands can be divided and trimmed back under local anaesthesia avoiding the urethra, anal canal and Bartholin's gland ducts. More complete barriers require specialist help and general anaesthesia
- *perineal sensitivity* following episiotomy or tear
- *vaginal dryness* commonly follows the menopause and can be treated by using vaginal lubricants during intercourse. Vaginal moisturisers and topical oestrogens are listed in the appropriate section in *Chapter 2*. Not allowing sufficient time for physiological lubrication to develop is a common cause of dyspareunia
- *vaginismus* is often considered a sign associated with psychosexual distress. Sensitive inquiry is essential as prior sexual abuse may be implicated. There appears to be some link between vaginismus and difficulty with relaxation during digital and speculum examination. Specialist psychosexual counselling can dramatically transform some couples' lives. See 'psychosexual difficulties' below
- *vulvar vestibulitis* and other vulval disorders, see below

Deep dyspareunia

As its name implies deep dyspareunia is felt deep within the pelvis and apart from ovulation sensitivity and traumatic intercourse may imply a pathological cause. Dyspareunia during and for some hours after intercourse is commonly reported. The treatments are dependent on aetiology. A low threshold for referral for secondary care opinion is recommended:

- *adenomyosis* or 'endometriosis interna' affects the myometrium. See below

- *cervicitis* may respond to cervical diathermy; refer
- *endometriosis* can cause dyspareunia depending on its location. See below
- *ovarian sensitivity* either related to the ovarian cycle or because an ovary lies in the pouch of Douglas 'in the line of fire'. Sexual technique and position can modify such problems. In persistent cases referral for consideration of laparoscopic treatment can be offered
- *pelvic adhesions* from previous surgery can restrict uterovaginal movement during coitus. The venous congestion that occurs during coitus causes pain in such instances. Seek specialist advice if this appears likely
- *pelvic inflammatory disease* renders the affected areas sensitive to the venous engorgement and mechanical effects of coitus
- *psychological disorder* is not a common cause of deep dyspareunia
- *retroversion of the uterus* is an occasional cause although most women with uterine retroversion have no problems. Pathological causes of retroversion should be considered (endometriosis, adhesions). Laparoscopic verterosuspension can be considered
- *traumatic intercourse* can obviously cause pain and even damage. Lacerations of the vagina and even through the fornices have been reported
- *vaginal infection* is a common transient cause

Ectopic pregnancy

Ectopic pregnancy most commonly occurs in the fallopian tube (95%). It can however occur adhering to pelvic viscera, the ovary, the uterine cornua and even the cervix. Only rarely are such pregnancies viable and ongoing (0.3% proceed to normal birth). Catastrophic life-threatening haemorrhage is the big danger and thus all suspected cases need immediate referral for specialist help. Ectopic pregnancy crops up significantly in each triennial Maternal Mortality Report, accounting for around 10% of cases.

Women having one ectopic gestation have at least a 1:3 chance of becoming pregnant again. Those who do conceive have a recurrent ectopic rate of up to 10%.

Predispositions to ectopic gestation

These include:

- *IUD contraception* does not cause ectopic gestation, in fact it reduces risk. However, because it prevents intrauterine pregnancy very effectively, breakthrough pregnancies are more likely to be the unprevented ectopic ones. Assume pregnancies with an IUD in situ are ectopic until proved otherwise
- *pelvic inflammatory disease* by damaging the fallopian tube. Even patent tubes may have endothelial damage interfering with oocyte transport
- *progestogen-only pill contraception* As with the IUD breakthrough, pregnancies are more likely to be ectopic. Assume POP pregnancies are ectopic until proved otherwise
- *race* Ectopic gestation is far more common among women of Afro-Caribbean ancestry
- *tubal surgery* because of the pre-existing damage (usually caused by pelvic infection) and scarring and adhesions that can complicate surgery

Presentation

This is as follows:

- **timing** is usually around 5–6 weeks gestation
- **pain** is the classic presentation. It may not be well localised laterally
- **tenderness** may be elicited on abdominal palpation
- **adnexal mass** may be encountered in an asymptomatic woman in early pregnancy. If encountered, on no account should it be palpated further

ABSOLUTE CONTRAINDICATION

Performance of vaginal examination in a woman strongly suspected of having an ectopic gestation is absolutely contraindicated unless it is done in an operating theatre with an anaesthetist present.

Management

Refer all cases to gynaecologist stat. No place for primary care management

Endometriosis

Endometriosis is a disorder caused by the presence of ectopic functioning endometrial tissues. The symptoms and consequences of ectopic endometrial cell deposits derive from their ability to respond to the hormonal changes of the ovarian cycle which result in repetitive ectopic menstruation. It is commonest among European and nulliparous women.

Aetiology is not fully elucidated but ideas include, retrograde menstruation, implantation at operation (eg. Caesarean section), vascular spread, cellular metaplasia. More than one mechanism may apply. There is also a familial link.

Terminology

- **adenomyosis**: ectopic endometrium within the uterine myometrium. Produces a bulky tender uterus, dysmenorrhoea and menorrhagia. Often first diagnosed after hysterectomy by the pathologist
- **chocolate cyst**: a pseudocyst containing altered blood and usually surrounded by dense fibrosis. A sign of advanced and usually severe disease. Chocolate cysts occur on the ovary and pelvic viscera. They can rupture and undergo torsion
- **endometrioma**: a mass of ectopic endometrial tissue usually with chocolate cyst development

- **endometriosis externa**: endometriotic deposits outside the uterus. Most commonly on ovary and uterosacral ligaments, but can involve urinary and GI tract. Distant deposits, for example in scars, in the umbilicus and even in lung or brain are reported
- **endometriosis interna**: another name for adenomyosis
- **pseudomenopause**: a form of treatment that stops the production of ovarian hormones.
- **pseudopregnancy**: a form of treatment that suppresses endometrial activity

- **stromal endometriosis**: an uncommon form of endometriosis and more resistant to treatment with solid masses of cells resembling endometrial stroma. Some histological features resemble malignancy. It peaks at 35–50 years of age, does not respond to oophorectomy and metastatic spread has been described

Clinical situations

deep dyspareunia

Deep dyspareunia almost always indicates pathology especially if it is a new development.

infertility

This is associated with endometriosis. Which causes which is not clear. Even tiny pelvic deposits reduce fertility. More advanced disease causes macroscopic pelvic damage which reduces fertility further.

non-genital manifestations

These include tenesmus with colonic involvement, urinary symptoms with ureteric involvement, and a number of less common symptoms like umbilical menstruation and cyclical haemoptysis. Chronic disease must also be a considerable emotional strain.

pelvic pain

Pelvic pain is commonly mentioned by women with endometriosis in addition to dysmenorrhoea and dyspareunia. Pressure sensations are also mentioned frequently.

reactivation of endometriosis

This can occur when oestrogen-containing HRT regimens are used. HRT must be used very cautiously, and with frequent reviews in women with a past history of endometriosis.

secondary dysmenorrhoea

Secondary dysmenorrhoea is always a pathological symptom and endometriosis is a classic cause. 'Crescendo' dysmenorrhoea is typical.

Therapeutic options

Because formal diagnosis will usually involve gynaecological opinions treatments are almost always initiated by secondary care specialists. Usual treatments are listed in *Table 1.6* and summarised below:

- *pseudopregnancy regimes* using continuous high dose progestogens
- *pseudomenopause regimes* result from pituitary down regulation using high dose danazol, gestrinone or gonadotrophin releasing hormone analogues (GnRH / LHRH analogues). The development of add back therapy has considerably improved the acceptability of GnRH therapy. Oestrogen, in the form of HRT, can be given alongside Zoladex to reduce the incidence of vasomotor symptoms which can complicate GnRH therapy. The reduction in bone mineral density is also significantly reduced. Any oestrogen HRT can be used, the choice being with the prescriber and the patient. It is important to choose a progestogen opposed product in non-hysterectomised women. Add back therapy can be continued for as long as the GnRH is required.
- *testosterone implants* can be used in women who have had a hysterectomy and where ovaries have not been removed

- **surgery** to assess and stage disease and allow removal of macroscopic deposits. Laparoscopy is particularly useful, allowing diathermy and laser ablation of deposits
- **support** is essential in this chronic painful condition that can produce involuntary infertility (support group address listed below)
- **others**: clomiphene, selenium ACE, Vitamin B6, evening primrose oil

Table 1.6: Treatments available for endometriosis

Drug treatments
Combined oral contraceptive pill: continuous therapy No pill-free intervals until breakthrough bleeding occurs. One of the more androgenic monophasic pills would be suitable (see COCP section of contraception chapter for side-effects, interactions etc)
Dydrogesterone: Tabs: 10 mg. Dose: 10 mg BD/TDS Cautions: diabetes, hypertension, cardiac and renal disease Contraindications: pregnancy, severe liver disease, severe arterial disease, breast and genital tract malignancy Side-effects: weight gain, acne, breast and libido changes, menstrual irregularity, PMS symptoms, depression, jaundice Interactions: rifampicin accelerates metabolism of progestogens; cyclosporin concentration increased
Medroxyprogesterone acetate: Tabs: 2 mg; 5 mg; 10 mg. Dose: 10 mg BD/TDS Cautions: side-effects etc as per didrogesterone
Norethisterone: Tabs: 5 mg. Dose: 5 mg TDS/QDS Cautions: side-effects etc as per didrogesterone
Danazol: Caps: 100 mg; 200 mg. Usual dose: 200 mg/day for 4–6 months (max dose 800 mg/day) Cautions: cardiac, renal or liver impairment, polycythaemia, diabetes Contraindications: pregnancy, lactation, thromboembolic disorder Side-effects: weight gain, acne, nausea, dizziness, defeminisation, virilisation Interactions: anticoagulant effects enhanced; carbamazepine and cyclosporin concentrations increased
Gestrinone: Caps: 2.5 mg. Dose: 2.5 mg twice weekly for 6 months Cautions: side-effects etc as per danazol
Testosterone implants: A secondary care option
GnRH/LHRH analogues: A secondary care option They are marketed as implants (Zoladex), injections (Prostap SR) and nasal sprays (Suprecur, Synarel). Side-effects mimic the climacteric. Prolonged therapy (>6 months) causes osteopaenia. Breakthrough bleeding can occur. The development of add back therapy has improved the situation for women with endometriosis who need GnRH therapy. See text

Useful address

The Endometriosis Society, 35 Belgrave Square, London, SW1X 8QB

Fibroids

Uterine fibroids are benign leiomyomas and are frequently asymptomatic. They occur more frequently in women of Afro-Caribbean origin. They usually distort the uterus but when they originate near either the endometrial or the serosal surfaces they can become pedunculate. Luminal fibroids may bulge or be extruded through the cervical canal into the vagina. Serosal pedunculate fibroids can tort, compress adjacent structures or become 'parasitic' on another structure.

Clinical situations

- **compression** of nearby viscera, particularly the bladder, can occur with large and small fibroids depending on the location

- **contraception** using the IUD is contraindicated if the uterine cavity is enlarged or distorted by fibroids. Oestrogens in the combined pill can promote the growth of fibroids

- **infertility** is said to be a rare consequence of fibroids. Perhaps more common is recurrent miscarriage which may very occasionally result particularly if the fibroids are submucous. Implantation and placentation over such a fibroid could result in placental insufficiency. Myomectomy and fibroid polypectomy is occasionally indicated

- **malignant transformation** complicates less than 1% of cases of uterine fibroids. Sarcomatous change may be marked by vaginal bleeding and pelvic pain. Rapid enlargement of a fibroid should raise suspicion of malignant change. Leiomyosarcomas are unrelated to parity and peak in women from the mid-forties to the mid-fifties

- **menopause** is usually followed by shrinking of fibroids, which are oestrogen-dependent benign tumours. If fibroids are present, oestrogen-containing HRT formulations should be used cautiously with regular bimanual assessment, as such formulations can stimulate the growth of fibroids

- **menorrhagia** caused by an increase in endometrial surface area and interference with haemostatic mechanisms is not uncommon with fibroids

- **pain,** especially during menstruation, is not uncommon. Dyspareunia may also occur

- **pregnancy** can be complicated by the presence of fibroids. Implantation over a submucous fibroid can lead to placental insufficiency and large submucous and cervical fibroids can cause dystocia (very rare). A more common event is red degeneration of fibroids. The hormones of pregnancy promote rapid fibroid growth which outstrips the vascular supply. The result is avascular necrosis which produces tenderness, pain and uterine irritability. Constitutional upset may occur. Myomectomy scars can rupture during pregnancy

- **urinary function** can be affected by fiboids either by compression of the bladder due to their size, or by distortion of the bladder base by low anterior or cervical fibroids

Therapeutic options

- **conservative management** is appropriate in three situations, namely: if the fibroids are asymptomatic; if the menopause is near and if their clinical impact is less than that of the therapeutic options. In some instances it may be appropriate to seek a second opinion to allow conservative management to be offered more confidently, especially if the fibroids are large and always if rapid growth occurs (sarcomatous change)

- **medical management** in primary care consists of treatment of the symptoms caused by the fibroid(s), eg. NSAIDs and iron for menorrhagia, and removal of drugs that promote their growth (the combined pill and HRT). In secondary care GnRH drugs can be used to shrink fibroids. Because regrowth frequently occurs after treatment and because they demineralise bone they are generally used as a preoperative or pre-pregnancy measure. There is evidence that the levonorgestrel intrauterine system (LNG-IUS, Mirena) causes some regression of uterine fibroids

- **surgical management** involves either removal of the fibroid (myomectomy) or removal of the uterus. Fibroid polyps and intra-abdominal pedunculate fibroids may be removed leaving the uterus intact. Myomectomy is performed when hysterectomy is contraindicated (patients' wishes, retention of fertility, operative difficulty). Myomectomy scars can rupture during pregnancy. Small submucous fibroids (<5 cm) can be removed or resected hysteroscopically

Hirsutism

Hair undergoes growth during anagen, involutes during catagen and rests during telogen. All hairs are associated with a sebaceous gland, hence the link between hirsutism and acne. Both structures are androgen sensitive. Once a hair is stimulated to produce terminal hair by androgens it will do so irrespective of the androgen level until after the next telogen phase.

Classification

A classification is listed below. This is a subject of massive endocrinological complexity. There is much interplay between the hormonal function of the ovary, the adrenal, peripheral fat and the production and effects of insulin resistance:

- **constitutional:** women who come from families that are endowed with more body hair than is perceived usual (avoiding the word normal) have more hair on the sideburns, chest, abdomen and legs. Ethnic factors, eg. women originating from the Mediterranean fringe, who have darker and more obvious hair are more physiologically hirsute than northern European women

- **cosmetic pressure** has made many normal women feel that they are not normal. Social pressures can be a source of distress in the absence of disease

- **drugs**: obviously androgens and anabolic steroids, which are increasingly drugs of misuse among sports women, can masculinise. Androgenic progestogens (norethisterone and levonorgestrel) in some combined contraceptive pills;

phenytoin, danazol and minoxidil can all have the same effect

- **ovarian causes** include polycystic ovary syndrome, ovarian tumour and hyperthecosis (rare). The theca is the LH driven functional part of the ovary and is distinct from the FSH driven oestrogen producing granulosa

- **adrenal causes**: adrenal hyperplasia can present in childhood or be a late onset problem. Adrenal tumours and Cushing's syndrome are causes
- **hyperprolactinaemia**
- **other factors** include obesity, hypothyroidism and the anovulatory state itself

---

Clinical situations

adrenal hyperplasia

This can present as a severe illness in infancy or childhood. A late onset variety can be asymptomatic or present with hirsutism in adult life. This common condition (it is an autosomal recessive disorder more common than cystic fibrosis) results from a 21-hydroxylase deficiency and results in a raised level of 17-hydroxyprogesterone. It can cause a costisol deficiency under stress conditions. The modest androgen and progesterone excess can be controlled by a small nightly dose of dexamethasone.

defeminisation/masculinisation

Defeminisation/masculinisation in association with excess body hair requires urgent secondary care investigation. Defeminisation describes oligomenorrhoea and breast atrophy. This is a normal response to oestrogen withdrawal and is often physiological, eg. the menopause. Masculinisation or virilism is, however, never physiological (except in multiple gestation pregnancy). The androgenic features include male pattern baldness, cliteromegally and deepening of the voice. Acne may also be a feature.

menstrual disturbance

Menstrual disturbance and hirsutism are closely linked. The polycystic ovary syndrome complex can induce both. Around 85% of women with oligomenorrhoea and hirsutism have PCOS. However, not all women with PCOS will be hirsute, obese and manifest acne. See below.

obesity and hirsutism

The links appear to be via reduced levels of the carrier protein SHBG allowing more testosterone to be unbound and active. This is especially evident in anovulatory women. Insulin resistance is also implicated. Weight loss can restore ovulation, allows SHBG to rise and free T to fall. A BMI of around $21Kg/m^2$ is the goal.

Investigations

Obviously these include a full history and examination. Hirsutism scoring charts such as the Ferriman and Gallway Charts (1961) are useful. Examination requires a detailed gynaecological and abdominal examination and a BMI score. The basic endocrine tests include FSH, LH, SHBG, testosterone, androstenedione, prolactin, 17-hydroxyprogesterone and thyroid function. More detailed tests, some of which involve measuring responses to ACTH challenges, are appropriate at the secondary/tertiary care level.

If inappropriate defeminisation or virilisation is evident urgent referral is mandatory. CT or MRI imaging of ovary and adrenals is necessary.

Treatments

Treatments are often effective but, with the exception of mechanical hair-removal, are slow. Hair follicles in telogen must have androgen drive removed before hirsutism can begin to respond. Anagen hairs have to be dropped at catagen:

- **androgen suppression** with the combined contraceptive pill will reduce androgenic effects. It also raises SHBG. Choose a pill with less androgenic progestogen (ie. avoiding norethisterone and levonorgestrel). See *Table 3.1* and *3.2*, pages 84 and 85. Dianette contains a very small dose of the anti-androgen cyproterone acetate (dose 2 mg)

- **anti-androgens**: The commonest drug is cyproterone acetate, which given in a reversed sequential schedule, is effective. The regime is ethinyloestradiol 30–50 mcg for 21 days combined with cyproterone acetate 50–100 mg for the first ten days of oestrogen treatment. It is repeated with seven-day pill free breaks. Spironolactone also blocks androgen receptors. A dose of 100–200 mg daily may be given. Eden (1991) recommends that it be given alongside a combined contraceptive pill. Regular electrolyte checks are required. Both cyproterone and spironolactone can feminise a male fetus. Treatment is generally continued for 6–12 months. Growth of hair often recurs slowly after treatment is stopped

- **dexamethasone** in small doses is very effective for proven 21-hydroxylase deficiency-induced hirsutism (0.05–0.25 mg nocte). Check others in the family as this is an autosomal recessive condition

- **hair removal:** shaving, waxing, bleaching and by electrolysis are often cosmetically effective

- **weight** is implicated in the endocrinological circuits of oestrogen, androgen, gonadotrophin and insulin activity. Weight reduction can restore ovulation, increase SHBG, reduce free testosterone, reduce insulin resistance and reduce LH levels. All will reduce the follicular drive to produce dark terminal hair. Aim at a BMI around 21Kg/m^2

References:

Eden JA (1991) Hirsutism. In: Studd J ed. *Progress in Obstetrics and Gynaecology,* Vol 9. Churchill Livingstone, Edinburgh

Ferriman D, Gallway JD (1961) Clinical assessment of body hair in women. *J Clin Endocrinol Metab* **21**: 1440–7

Infection

Actinomycosis

This is covered in the IUD section of *Chapter 3*.

Bacterial vaginosis

This has been listed individually above.

Candidiasis

Candidiasis is listed individually above.

Chlamydia

This is frequently a sexually transmitted disease with the ability to cause silent upper genital tract (particularly fallopian tube) damage. Referral to a specialist in genito-urinary medicine rather than initiating treatment in the primary care setting is strongly advised.

Gonorrhoea

Gonorrhoea is almost exclusively a sexually transmitted disease and should always prompt referral to a GUMed specialist. One STD is frequently contracted along with others. Appropriate swabs and samples will have to be taken to exclude other infections.

Herpes simplex virus infection

This can be a sexually transmitted infection, but can also be transmitted by auto-inoculation from 'cold sores'.

HIV

HIV is discussed in relation to pregnancy in *Chapter 6*, to lactation in *Chapter 8* and in relation to the IUD in *Chapter 3*. It is not discussed further here.

HPV

HPV causes genital warts (condyloma accuminata) and is usually contacted through sexual contact although there is evidence for vertical transmission from the mother at birth. Several serotypes are implicated in the oncogenesis of cervical and vulval carcinoma. Although macroscopic warts can be treated with application of liquid nitrogen or podophyllin the viral particles seeded in the epithelial 'field' will not be removed. Women with genital warts require specialist genito-urinary care.

Mycoplasma hominis

This is thought to cause some cases of post abortal sepsis. Its role as a pathogen otherwise is not clear and although it may be transmissible sexually it is not known whether it is exclusively transmitted in this way.

Toxic shock syndrome

Toxic shock syndrome is discussed separately in a later section.

Trichomonas vaginalis

This disease is almost exclusively sexually transmitted and should always prompt referral to a GUMed specialist. One STD is frequently contracted along with others. Appropriate swabs and samples will have to be taken to exclude other infections.

Ureaplasma urealyticum

This is a chlamydia/mycoplasma like organism. It is thought to cause some cases of post abortal sepsis but, apart from this, its role as a pathogen is unclear. Although it may be transmissible sexually it is not known whether it is exclusively transmitted in this way.

Intraepithelial neoplasia

Although intraepithelial neoplasia can develop in all epithelial surfaces of the lower genital tract, the cervix and vulva are the areas of principal clinical concern.

Cervical intraepithelial neoplasia (CIN)

This is a histological diagnosis obtained from tissue biopsy specimens. Biopsy is usually prompted by the finding of dyskaryotic cytological abnormality on cervical smear tests. The human papilloma virus is implicated, indeed, research on the value of screening for the virus itself as a pointer towards the presence of CIN is underway. The mildest dysplastic features (CIN I) have considerable histological overlap with those of HPV infection. CIN can be a precursor to squamous cell carcinoma of the cervix.

clinical questions

- *abnormal smear results in pregnancy* require expert colposcopic investigation. Biopsies may need to be taken despite the increased risk of haemorrhage in pregnancy. If a recent smear test report is not available a smear should be taken in early pregnancy. A balance has to be struck between the consequence to the fetus of cervical procedures or even early delivery and the urgency for treatment of the disease, if invasive cancer has developed. A tertiary care problem

- *adenocarcinoma of the cervix* is far less common than squamous carcinoma. It can be detected on cervical smears. Glandular atypia on a report requires referral to a gynaecologist/colposcopist. Incidence may be increasing in younger women

- *clinical associations*: the classic demographic and behavioural associations are early first intercourse, multiple sexual partners, non-barrier contraception, past history of STD, cigarette smoking and of course HPV infection

- *diethylstilboestrol exposure* in utero increases risks in girls to clear cell vaginal carcinoma as well as cervical and vaginal dysplasia

- *HIV and CIN* are associated strongly. In the United States, women whose CIN recurs rapidly after primary treatment are now offered HIV pre-test counselling and screening

- *individual screening* and whether it should be more frequent than the community programmes recommend. The marginally improved pick up rate (which is not the same as prevention of cancer — the whole point, after all, of screening) has to be balanced against the cost implications to the community and the increase in the number of false positive results, with the attendant implications for the individual being screened (colposcopy, cervical biopsy, anxiety etc)

- *population screening* is recommended, especially for the high risk women who are least likely to attend. Improving the screen by reducing false positive (currently around 5%) and false negative results using cervical photography and incorporating HPV DNA assays into the screen are under way

- *virgins* are not immune to CIN and cervical cancer. The classical paper 'Nuns, virgins and spinsters. Rigorni Stern and cervical cancer revisited' by M Griffith argued that although their risk was lower than in their non-celibate sisters it was still significant. Cervical cytological screening should be offered to all women with a cervix

Vulval intraepithelial neoplasia (VIN)

This is a histological diagnosis obtained from tissue biopsy specimens. Biopsy is usually prompted by the complaint of vulval symptoms or the finding of vulval skin abnormalities. VIN is strongly associated with the presence of HPV infection and can be a precursor to squamous carcinoma of the vulva. Always refer to a gynaecologist with a particular interest in VIN and colposcopy.

clinical questions

- **Clinical associations** include HPV infection, CIN, perianal pre-malignancy and malignancy. The classic demographic and behavioural associations are early first intercourse, multiple partners, low socio-economic status, past history of STD, past history of abnormal cervical smear and cigarette smoking

- **diagnosis** is made histologiocally from biopsy specimens. VIN is frequently multifocal and several biopsies may be required. If VIN is diagnosed, refer to a gynaecologist

- **progression rates** to invasive cancer in the untreated are quoted at around 20% over a ten-year period

- **vulval symptoms and skin change** should always be taken seriously. For those capable, a biopsy is the diagnostic test. If there are doubts about vulval skin anomalies a dermatological or gynaecological referral should be made. See vulval disorder, below

Vaginal intraepithelial neoplasia (VAIN)

VAIN may be noticed during colposcopic examination of the cervix. Six percent of women with CIN will have VAIN. Its management is usually at the tertiary level. Vaginal adenosis and VAIN are more common in women exposed to DES *in utero*.

Reference

Griffith M (1991) Nuns, virgins and spinsters. Rigorni Stern and cervical cancer revisited. *Br J Obstet Gynaecol* **98**: 797–802

Labial adhesion

Congenital types

Congenital types are uncommon and may be a manifestation of ambiguous external genitalia. Tertiary opinions may be required.

Childhood

In childhood, during the years of 'oestrogen lack', labial adhesion can develop spontaneously. It usually responds to the application of topical oestrogen cream. Short term use is all that is required. Systemic or uterine absorption can result in a withdrawal bleed at the end of treatment. This is of no clinical significance and parents who have not been forewarned can be reassured. Episodes of vulvovaginitis in childhood can also cause adhesion and should alert the attendant to the possibility of sexual abuse. It is possible for foreign bodies (beads, clothing fragments) and occasionally threadworms to be the seat of infection in children.

After childbirth

After childbirth, episiotomy and tears can produce adhesions as a result of healing and repair. Small surgical procedures may be required although minor adhesions which cause dyspareunia can, with care and gentleness, stretch up nicely without the need for recourse to surgery.

Postmenopausal adhesions

These may develop as part of the atrophy process.

Menstrual disturbance

Disorders of menstruation are exceedingly common comprising one fifth of gynaecology referrals and accounting for the majority of the one in five women who have had a hysterectomy by the age of 55 years. At some stage, 22% of women will complain of menorrhagia. Probably the greatest challenge for the primary care management of menstrual disturbance is in the rationalisation of progestogen prescribing.

Terminology

- **amenorrhoea**: cessation of menstruation for six months or more
- **cryptomenorrhoea** describes menstruation that is not expelled from the body. It can be primary (eg. as a result of congenital atresia or imperforate hymen) or secondary (eg. stenosis following cervical surgery). Both are rare
- **DUB**: dysfunctional uterine bleeding is menstrual disturbance in the absence of pregnancy, infection, tumour or bleeding diathesis
- **menarche**: first menstrual period
- **menopause**: the final menstrual period
- **menorrhagia:** subjective reporting of heavy periods. Objective finding of total menstrual blood loss greater than 80 ml per period

- **metropathia haemorrhagica**: excessive menstruation at long intervals associated with avovulation and cystic glandular hyperplastic change in the endometrium (Swiss cheese pattern)
- **metrorrhagia**: irregular vaginal bleeding between periods. Synonymous with intermenstrual bleeding
- **oligomenorrhoea**: menstrual cycles between six weeks and six months
- **PMB**: postmenopausal bleeding should be considered in any climacteric or postmenopausal women more than six months past their last normal menstrual period
- **polymenorrhoea**: a menstrual cycle of less than twenty-one days

Clinical situations:

intermenstrual bleeding

This has a wide variety of possible causes, all of which should be considered in women presenting with it. Post coital bleeding may have similar causes:

- ***cervical causes*** must always be excluded. Cervical polyps, cervical erosion and although uncommon, cervical carcinoma

- **drugs**, especially contraceptive steroids, must be considered. Drugs that interact with contraceptive steroids can also lead to irregular endometrial shedding
- **endometrial causes** are common. Erratic shedding of endometrium can occur spontaneously or as a complication of contraceptive pill use. Endometrial polyps may also cause intermenstrual bleeding
- **ovulation** is said to be associated occasionally with a mid-cycle 'show'. Beware missing pathology because metrorrhagia may occur mid-cycle
- **pregnancy** must always be considered as a spurious cause of intermenstrual loss

menorrhagia

Menorrhagia is often diagnosed on the subjective experiences of women. Correlation between the perception of the heaviness of menstrual loss and the actual volume passed per cycle is poor. It is generally considered that menstrual blood loss in excess of 80 ml per cycle will lead to depletion of iron stores. In the literature this is used to define the threshold for menorrhagia. Precise measurement requires haematin elution from sanitary wear which is clinically impractical. However, charts for assessing MBL by the number and heaviness of soiling of sanitary wear can be used in primary care to aid diagnosis and measure the effects of treatment (Jasson *et al*, 1995). Treatments are listed in *Table 1.7*.

The causes of excessive menstruation are:

- **bleeding disorders** are rare causes of menorrhagia. A normal clotting screen and platelet count will often reassure
- **dysfunctional bleeding** is defined as abnormal menstrual blood loss in the absence of pregnancy, infection, organic pathology (fibroids, endometrial carcinoma) and bleeding diathesis. It is thought to occur either because progesterone production is inadequate or absent or because of prostaglandin production at the level of the endometrium
- **endometriosis** is a well known cause of menorrhagia and is usually associated with congestive dysmenorrhoea, dyspareunia and involuntary infertility
- **infection** in the pelvic viscera can mimic endometriotic symptoms
- **IUDs** with the exception of the levonogestrel intrauterine system (Mirena) lead to heavier and longer MBL. If unacceptable or resistant to treatment removal may be the only option
- **pregnancy** should always be considered as a spurious cause of menstrual problems. A rarity related to pregnancy is trophoblastic disease
- **tumour**: uterine fibroids can increase the endometrial surface area and by distorting the uterus interfere with haemostasis. Uterine fibroid polyps are a variation on this theme. From the age of about forty, especially in the obese, the possibility of endometrial carcinoma should be considered, although this is much more common in the post-menopausal years.

metropathia haemorrhagica

This is the result of unopposed exposure of the endometrium to oestrogen. The histological consequence is endometrial cystic glandular hyperplasia (the Swiss cheese pattern). The clinical consequences are infrequent, unpredictable, heavy but usually painless menorrhagia. The causes of it are:

- **anovulation** which is physiological at menarche and in the climacteric. No ovulation means no progesterone and so no opposition of oestrogen. Treatment with progestogens to cause a secretory change in the endometrium is effective

- **drugs** in the form of unopposed oestrogens could cause metropathia. Continual use of the combined pill without breaks is different because progestogens are contained in their formulation
- **polycystic ovary syndrome** can cause metropathia because of anovulation. Most women with PCOS do not exhibit the classical Stein-Leventhal picture of obesity and hirsutism. See below.

oligomenorrhoea

Oligomenorrhoea may be a physiological variation or signify anovulation. Rarely the cause may lie in the pituitary (eg. prolactinoma) or hypothalamus (eg. stress, anorexia nervosa) or be the result of excess androgen secretion. Androgens, in these cases, come from hyperplastic adrenals or ovarian tumours and may cause oligomenorrhoea in a defeminising phase before virilisation develops. Diagnosis is made from history and examination, supplemented by assaying pituitary gonadotrophins (FSH and LH), prolactin and, if appropriate, oestradiol and testosterone. The endocrinological work up for adrenal hyperplasia is a tertiary care problem. Refer urgently any cases of suspected defeminisation or virilisation:

- **physiological**: the limits of the normal range are open ended. Menstruation may be infrequent without being caused by anything other than the imperfect and variable human condition
- **androgenic causes** of oligo/amenorrhoea are rare. A defeminising phase may make menstruation infrequent before amenorrhoea and masculinisation develops. Adrenal hyperplasia and ovarian tumours are the usual sources of excess androgens. The endocrinological work up for adrenal hyperplasia is a tertiary care problem. Refer urgently any cases of suspected defeminisation or virilisation
- **anovulation,** as discussed above, under metropathia heamorrhagica is a cause of oliomenorrhoea
- **drugs** can interfere with ovulation. Depot progestogens and implants are obvious as is danazol. Take a drug history and, if appropriate, enquire about illicit use of body building anabolic steroids
- **hypothalamic causes** include stress and general debility and, of course, anorexia nervosa and low body weight. The pituitary gonadotrophins are low in such instances
- **ovarian causes** include ovarian senescence (climacteric) and ovarian resistance. Pituitary gonadotrophins will be raised in both instances
- **pituitary causes** must be considered of which a pituitary adenoma (prolactinoma) is the classic case (galactorrhoea/amenorrhoea syndrome). Check prolactin FSH and LH.

References

Jasson CA *et al* (1995) A simple visual assessment technique to discriminate between menorrhagia and normal menstrual blood loss. *Obstet Gynecol* **85**: 977–82

Lahteenmaki P *et al* (1998) Open randomised study of levonorgestrel releasing intrauterine system as an alternative to hysterectomy. *Br Med J* **316**: 1122–6

Table 1.7: Treatments available for menorrhagia

Drug	Regime	Notes
combined pill	as for contraception	very effective measure, shortened or less frequent pill free intervals improves effect
NSAIDs	Ibuprofen 400 mg tds naproxen 250 mg tds mefenamic acid 500 mg tds	inhibit prostaglandin metabolism and so reduce uterine cramps and MBL. More effective if commenced one or two days before period begins but caution required if any chance of pregnancy. Beware also of use in dyspeptics and asthmatics
tranexamic acid	1 g tds during period	an underused antifibrinolytic which does not cause thrombotic strokes as some isolated case reports suggested. The most consistently effective treatment in clinical trials
ethamsylate	500 mg qds during menstruation	also underused drug reduces capilliary fragility and inhibits prostacycline synthetase
danazol	100 mg/day x 3 months	very effective in the short term, beware side-effects even at low dose
Mirena IUS	intrauterine device	licensed for contraception but reduces MBL dramatically in most women. 20% amenorrhoeic at end of first year*
aspirin		ineffective
progestogens	norethisterone 5mg tds dydrogesterone 10 mg bd medroxyprogesterone acetate 2.5–10 mg/day in divided doses	trials have, however, only looked at luteal phase use, eg. day 16–21 or day 19–26. Clinical experience with day 5–15 usage suggests progestogens are beneficial. Use of progestogens in this way is, however, only a short term option. Far better therapies are now available

* One recent study showed measurable benefit in a group of women with severe menstrual problems. For the present the IUS must be viewed as a cheap and safe but currently out of licence option in women with dysfunctional uterine bleeding. It certainly carries a far lower morbidity, mortality and economic burden than hysterectomy and should be added to the list of other treatment options for DUB (Lahteenmaki P. 1998)

Miscarriage (abortion)

Miscarriage is defined here as the ending of pregnancy by whatever means prior to its 24th week. The term 'abortion' has emotive connotations and 'miscarriage' is generally reserved for spontaneous abortions. Induced abortions can be legal (therapeutic), or criminal.

Terminology

- **blighted ovum** describes a non-viable pregnancy where no fetal pole is identifiable on ultrasonic scanning or when the products of conception are examined

- **complete miscarriage** is the spontaneous and total expulsion of the conception. Ultrasound confirmation of completion permits surgical evacuation to be avoided
- **criminal abortion** occurs when abortion is procured without strict adherence to the terms of the Abortion Act. Almost unheard of in the UK now, it was common before the introduction of the 1967 Act. Genital tract damage and sepsis were common complications with a significant morbidity and mortality
- **early miscarriage** occurs up to twelve weeks and is often the result of chromosomal anomaly in the fetus
- **habitual miscarriage** or recurrent miscarriage is defined when three or more consecutive spontaneous miscarriages occur. Even in this unhappy circumstance, the chance that a fourth pregnancy will miscarry is less than 1:2
- **incomplete miscarriage** is deemed to have occurred when some of the products of conception are not expelled. Bleeding, pain and sepsis are possible sequelae
- **induced miscarriage** occurs when intervention is made to terminate an otherwise ongoing pregnancy (see therapeutic abortion)
- **inevitable miscarriage** exists when a pregnancy is committed to miscarrying but the process is not yet complete. It is usually diagnosed when the cervical os is found to have opened
- **late miscarriage** occurs after the twelfth week. The later it occurs the more it resembles premature labour
- **legal abortion** is a procured or induced abortion performed in accordance with the Abortion Act
- **missed miscarriage** is diagnosed when a non-viable fetus is found in a pregnancy that has not started to miscarry spontaneously. It can be suspected if the uterine size is less than dates would suggest and if the symptoms of pregnancy have regressed
- **pregnancy reduction** may be considered in high grade multiple pregnancies, usually following problems with gonadotrophin ovulation induction. The take home baby rate is increased when, for example, sextuplets are reduced to twins. Reduced prematurity increases the 'quality' of the babies who survive. Reduction of a normal twin pregnancy to singleton however poses ethical questions and moral dilemmas and is more about social issues rather than the number and quality of babies ultimately taken home. 'Reduction' is achieved by killing the most conveniently placed fetuses usually with a maternal transabdominal fetal intracardiac injection. The conceptions involute rather than miscarry although loss of the entire pregnancy is a risk
- **recurrent miscarriage:** see habitual miscarriage
- **septic miscarriage** is usually minor but can be extremely serious so always requires admission. Uncontrolled infection can progress to endotoxic shock. It was formerly common after criminal abortion
- **spontaneous miscarriage** describes any miscarriage that occurs without being induced
- **therapeutic abortion** describes a legal, induced abortion
- **threatened miscarriage** is very common and is diagnosed when any bleeding from the genital tract occurs after the last normal menstrual period and before 24 weeks' gestation. Most settle. A proportion proceed to inevitability
- **tubal miscarriage** is an uncommon occurrence when a pregnancy dies in the fallopian tube. Expulsion is impossible. Involution occurs

Clinical situations

spontaneous miscarriage (early)

This occurs in 15% of pregnancies. No investigations are required for first or even second miscarriages. For three or more miscarriages treat as recurrent miscarriage. Management is aimed at:

- *diagnosis*: was the woman actually pregnant at all or is she experiencing a menstrual disturbance?
- *controlling pain*: in addition to usual analgesics which should be parenteral if surgical evacuation of the uterus is likely, clearing products of conception from the cervical os can dramatically reduce pain and bleeding
- *controlling bleeding*: evacuation of products from the os and ultimately completion of the miscarriage, either spontaneously or surgically, will control bleeding. Ergometrine, oxytocin and combinations of the two can be given to control heavy bleeding and to contract the uterus which normally occurs when the process is complete (see *Table 1.8*)
- *avoiding sepsis*: involves consideration of pre-existing factors, using sterile instruments and an aseptic technique and ensuring a swift and complete conclusion to the miscarriage process
- *facilitating emotional readjustment*: miscarriage is followed by varying degrees of grief for the lost potential. Shock, anger, guilt and readjustment are stages that may well be encountered. Most gynaecologists advise a delay of two or more months before trying to conceive again principally to allow the uterus to recover, but also to allow time for grieving to reach a conclusion. Many hospital units have close contact with miscarriage support groups (see useful addresses below)

Table 1.8: Drug treatments used in spontaneous miscarriage

Anti-D Immunoglobulin should be given to Rhesus-negative women who bleed in pregnancy to prevent the formation of anti-D antibodies. All pregnancies should be assumed to be Rh-D positive. The injection is available through local blood transfusion service departments and local arrangements will be in place for its delivery. The immunisation should be given within 72 hours of the bleeding event. Fetal blood cell counts in maternal peripheral blood (Kliehaur test) will indicate whether extra doses of anti-D I g are required

Ergometrine maleate tablets 500 mcg and injection 500 mcg/ml, I ml

Ergometrine maleate 500 mcg x Oxytocin 5 u/ml injection, Iml (Syntometrine) dose
Indication: control of haemorrhage in incomplete miscarriage
Cautions: cardiac disease, hypertension, liver or renal disorder, porphyria
Contraindications: labour I° and 2° stages of labour, severe cardiac failure, vascular disease, pulmonary disease, renal or liver disease, sepsis
Interactions: Erythromycin and azithromycin: risk of ergotism. Beta-blockers: peripheral vasoconstriction enhanced. Sumatriptan: risk of vasospasm increased

Oxytocin (Syntocinon): not applicable in primary care as it should be given by infusion

spontaneous miscarriage (late)

By the end of the twelfth week 90% of miscarriages will have occurred. The principals of treatment are similar to early miscarriage with some additions. The later in pregnancy the miscarriage occurs, the more it resembles preterm labour and, in general, the greater the distress and grief. The aetiology changes from being almost a 'normal abnormality' to one with clinical significance. Possibilities to consider include:

- ***fetal abnormality resulting in fetal death***
- ***uterine and cervical structural abnormalities*** (eg. cervical incompetence, bicornuate uterus)
- ***sepsis*** (CMV, bacterial vaginosis, listeriosis)
- ***multiple gestation***
- ***maternal medical conditions*** (eg. antiphospholipid antibodies, lupus anticoagulant, SLE)

It is important that the correct investigations are performed so that acute conditions like infection can be treated, a satisfactory explanation can be given to the family if possible about why the miscarriage has occurred and so that informed advice on planning future pregnancies can be given. This will involve emergency referral to a gynaecologist who will consider karyotyping the fetus and parents, screening for infection and atypical antibodies (some of which rapidly disappear after pregnancy) and perhaps arranging cervical resistance studies.

recurrent (habitual) abortion

This is generally considered where three or more consecutive spontaneous miscarriages have occurred. Even in this situation for a woman becoming pregnant for the fourth time the likelihood of achieving a live birth is 60%. Management considerations are as follows:

- ***chromosome anomaly*** should be considered. Karyotyping both parents and where possible fetal tissues from any subsequent miscarriages
- ***infection***: toxoplasma and mycoplasma can cause recurrent miscarriage
- ***maternal disease*** particularly autoimmune disorders should be screened for. It is also usual to check thyroid function and glucose levels. Miscarriage is more common in women who drink alcohol and caffeine drinks
- ***phospholipid antibodies***: around 15% of recurrent miscarriers have phospholipid antibodies, either lupus anticoagulant or anticardiolipid antibodies or both. Concurrent treatment with aspirin and heparin in pregnancy considerably improves the chances of a live birth. A secondary/tertiary care problem (Rai, R 1997)
- ***luteal phase deficiency***: the ovarian corpus luteum is a hormonal factory that supports the pregnancy until the placenta takes over at around 6–8 weeks. Progesterone has been used to support its function in a recurrent miscarrier. Progesterone deficiency has been diagnosed by examination of cytological preparations, vaginal skin scrapings and titrating the dose of progesterone accordingly (karyo-pyknotic index, KPI). Histological analysis of an LH timed endometrial biopsy has superseded the KPI. This is the remit of a specialist in fertility medicine
- ***support*** is obviously essential. Consider support groups.

threatened miscarriage

Around 90% of these pregnancies do not miscarry. Always consider non-pregnancy causes of bleeding of which cervical carcinoma, although rare, is the classical case. Always determine Rhesus antigen status; women who are Rh D negative should be given Anti-D immunoglobulin. Bed rest is commonly advised despite the lack of evidence that it is useful. Avoiding intercourse is also usually advised for a week or two.

therapeutic miscarriage

This is performed in over 120,000 women or one in five of all pregnancies in the UK each year (see sections on contraception and emergency contraception). In most cases it is performed for unwanted pregnancy. In some cases it is performed because of fetal anomaly or maternal illness.

In any case the terms of the Abortion Act must be complied with. Practitioners with ethical objections to termination of pregnancy are not obliged to arrange or take part in procuring abortion, but are duty bound after counselling to refer the women on to someone who will arrange it if the woman so wishes. Unco-operative and obstructive behaviour is unacceptable. Management involves consideration of:

- **exploration of the background** of the request for referral for termination of pregnancy. A straightforward request may in fact be a plea for support and assistance to continue with a pregnancy against the wishes of third parties
- **consideration of proceeding with the pregnancy** and opting for adoption; an option that is rarely exercised, but one that ought to be considered
- **consideration of medical termination** in women up to 63 days since the last period began. It involves administration of the anti-progestogen mifepristone (RU 486) in an approved unit, followed a few days later by a prostaglandin which causes the abortion. A proportion of cases subsequently require surgical evacuation of the uterus. The standard regime involves the administration of mifepristone followed by two hours of observation. Forty-eight hours later 1mg of gemprost is administered vaginally. Complete abortion occurs in 90% of cases and the ongoing pregnancy rate is less than 1%. A new lower dose regime has recently been introduced (mifepristone 200 mg followed forty-eight hours later by misoprostol 400 mcg pv) (Stewart P, 1996)
- **consideration of surgical termination** for women presenting later than 63 days or who prefer the method
- **advising about late termination options**: usually after 12 weeks (or earlier in nulliparous and very young women) suction evacuation may be inadvisable. Inducing a mini-labour with, for example, extra-amniotic prostaglandins or the less commonly performed dilatation and evacuation procedure should be sensitively discussed
- **follow up contraception** is usually of great importance and should always be considered as part of the follow through after therapeutic abortion
- **follow up support** is especially important where termination was performed because of fetal anomaly. The range of support groups is as broad as that of the possible pathologies. Specific groups may be contacted via the local gynaecology unit or through one of the broader agencies mentioned below
- **screening for genital tract pathogens** that may opportunistically cause post abortal sepsis is good practice and usually undertaken by the abortion service provider
- **Rhesus D negative women** should receive anti-D immunoglobulin injection at the time of the abortion.

References

Stewart P (1996) New indications for the use of Mifepristone and Misoprostol. *Trends Urol Gynaecol Sex Health* **1(4)**: 9–10

Rai R *et al* (1997) Randomised controlled trial of aspirin and aspirin plus heparin in pregnant women with recurrent miscarriage associated with phospholipid antibodies (or antiphospholipid antibodies). *Br Med J* **314**: 253–7

Useful addresses:

Miscarriage Association, c/o Claydon Hospital, Northgate, Wakefield WF1 3JS;
Tel: 01924 200799

Stillbirth and Neonatal Death Society (SANDS), 28 Portland Place, London W1N 4DE;
Tel: 0171 436 7940; Helpline: 0171 436 5881

Ovarian cyst

The ovary produces the largest range of neoplastic disorders in the human body. Ovarian growths can be solid, cystic or mixed. Some contain recognisable inappropriate tissue, eg. teeth in dermoids. Some secrete hormones and are rare causes of thyrotoxicosis and virilism. The ovary can be the host for metastatic tumour. All but the smallest solitary presumed functional ovarian cysts require a rapid gynaecological opinion. Even the most innocuous cysts require careful follow up. See 'Ovarian cancer' above and 'Screening for ovarian cancer' below.

Classification

- **functional**: during the fertile years the ovary regularly produces cysts that rupture (ovulation). Follicular and luteal cysts are common. They can be persistent and can be subject to accidents
- **endometriotic pseudocysts** can develop. The ovary is a frequent site for endometriosis
- **polycystic disease** produces numerous small peripheral cysts under a thickened capsule. See below
- **neoplastic cysts** are common. They are often asymptomatic. All should be referred on for ultrasonic scanning and further investigation:
  - benign
  - borderline
  - malignant
- **metastatic cancer** on the ovary, classically from breast and endometrial primaries
- **Woolfian remnant cysts** can develop within the broad ligament and inferior to the fimbrial end of the Fallopian tube

Clinical situations

- **asymptomatic ovarian** cysts should be referred for a gynaecological opinion. A small (<5cm), asymptomatic, single cyst that is found during a routine examination may be left for a month or six weeks. If it persists, however, referral should be arranged. Conservative management aided by ultrasonic scanning and CA 125 tumour marker measurement is a secondary care decision
- **compression** of surrounding structures. A rare cause of urinary retention
- **haemorrhage** into a cyst can cause an acute abdominal emergency
- **infection** within a cyst, presumably haematogenous spread can occur
- **rupture** can cause collapse and an acute abdomen. The main differential diagnosis is ruptured ectopic pregnancy
- **torsion** is another gynaecological emergency. Rapid intervention can save the ovary

Ovulation pain

Also known as Mittelschmerz. It is not clear whether the pain of ovulation is caused by rupture of the ovarian follicle and the release of fluid and a little blood onto the peritoneum or by the LH surge that precedes it by 24 hours. LH can increase perifollicular smooth muscle contractility mediated by prostaglandin F2α. It may be that both can cause pain. The experience of mid-cycle pain (more accurately two weeks prior to the next menstruation) suggests ovulation. It may be localised unilaterally. Excessive ovulation pain may be associated with peri-ovarian adhesions.

Treatment

- *analgesics* are usually appropriate. The NSAIDs may be more effective than paracetamol and codeine-based preparations
- *ovulation suppression* with the combined contraceptive pill. A depot progestogen can be considered in troublesome cases. The use of danazol or GnRH drugs would be difficult to justify. If they appeared to be needed one would have to question whether the diagnosis was correct (PID, endometriosis, pelvic mass etc)

Pelvic inflammatory disease

This term implies an ascending infection of the upper genital tract. More precision is required in both the use of the term and in the description of its manifestation in a particular individual. The presence of an infection, even gonococcus, does not mean PID has developed. PID may proceed subclinically.

Varieties of PID

Varieties of PID range from endometritis through parametritis to salpingitis and salpingo-oophoritis. Abscess development and pelvic peritonitis are serious developments. Precision in describing the mode of presentation is important.

Aetiology of PID

- *contraception*: either at the time of IUD fitting or subsequently (eg. A. Israelii)
- *iatrogenic infection* introduced at the time of performing a pelvic surgical procedure
- *sexual activity* is related to the development of upper genital tract infection. Vaginal flora may be mechanically transported up the cervical canal. There is evidence that motile spermatozoa and trichomonas organisms can carry microbes as they move up the cervical canal
- *sexually transmitted disease* is the most important area of concern:
  - *primary infection* may be with a classic STD like the gonococcus or with chlamydia trachomatis. It may be short lived and may not even cause the women to present to a health professional

- *secondary infection* following an initiating primary infection appears to be the main cause of PID. The primary infection sets the scene and allows a variety of opportunistic microbes (bacterioides, peptococci) to establish
- *recurrent and chronic disease*

Cardinal features of PID

- ***abdominal pain***, deep dyspareunia
- ***bilateral adnexal tenderness***
- ***cervical excitation*** (gentle lateral movement of the cervix provokes severe pain)
- ***pyrexia***
- ***vaginal discharge*** may be absent

Features related to sexually transmitted PID

These include:
- ***purulent vaginal discharge***
- ***a raised ESR*** >15mm/hour or the presence of leucocytosis
- ***gonococcus*** isolated on swabs or culture
- ***adnexal swelling***
- ***pyrexia*** >38°
- ***youth*** <25 years of age
- ***relationships***: less common among those in stable monogamous relationships

If a woman with lower abdominal pain has all seven risk factors the likelihood of PID is around 97%. If none are present the risk is around 7%.

Complications

These range from long term pelvic pain, dysmenorrhoea and dyspareunia to tubal damage and infertility. Pelvic peritonitis and abscess formation carries a small mortality risk.

Diagnosis

This is achieved ideally at laparoscopy. In the primary care setting the clinical features supplemented by microbiological testing can enable diagnosis. Swabs need to be recovered from the vagina, endocervix, urethra and include an endocervical swab specifically for chlamydia trachomatis. An MSU and FBC are useful.

Management

If there are any concerns about, for example, future fertility or if a sexually transmitted cause is suspected refer to a GUMed specialist. If pyrexia or a mass is present admission is recommended either under a GUMed physician or gynaecologist. Beware! Gynaecologists are essentially surgeons and may well omit to perform a full STD screen or arrange follow up and contact tracing. If a sexually transmitted cause is not suspected and in the presence of mild disease, it may be permissible to treat PID in primary care with antibiotics. The main pitfalls are missing sexually transmitted disease and, in particular, chlamydia which can silently cause continuing fallopian tube damage.

Treatment

Ideally, treatment should be under the care of a genitourinary physician. Occasionally, the primary care doctor will have to give treatment, eg. for a patient who absolutely refuses GUMed involvement or a patient who is unavoidably about to travel. Guidance on treatment should be sought from the local GUMed specialist.

In all cases the importance of adequate follow up after empirical treatment to 'test the cure' with appropriate microbiological investigation can hardly be stressed too greatly.

Prevention

Taking microbiological swabs prior to IUD insertion and before pelvic surgery can enable early or preventative therapy to be given. Screen for gonococcus, bacterial vaginosis, chlamydia trachomatis and mycoplasma. Ureaplasma may be an opportunist in such circumstances; research on this question is ongoing.

Pelvic pain syndrome

Chronic pelvic pain is a frequent complaint encountered in primary care. Because a diagnosis is rarely secured it often leads to frustration for both the sufferer and her attendant. Chronic pelvic pain accounts for more than half of all gynaecological diagnostic laparoscopies. Endometriosis is probably the most important condition in practice to avoid missing. The differential diagnoses include:

Gynaecological causes of chronic pelvic pain

- **endometriosis** classically produces pain, dysmenorrhoea, dyspareunia and infertility
- **neoplasia**
  - *benign*: large uterine fibroids and ovarian cyst
  - *malignant disease* of the genital tract
- **pelvic inflammatory disease** (PID) has many features in common with endometriosis
- **pelvic pain syndrome** (PPS): a diagnosis about which there is still hot debate. Commonest in the mid-reproductive years, this syndrome is said to be caused by pelvic venous congestion. It occurs more commonly on the left side although it may swap sides or be bilateral. It is associated with deep dyspareunia, post-coital discomfort and secondary dysmenorrhoea
- **adhesions** from previous pelvic surgery can cause chronic pelvic pain. Adhesions may, on the other hand, produce no ill effects at all. Characteristically, the adhesions that cause pelvic pain, which has its onset within a month or two of surgery, involve the parietal peritoneum, vaginal vault or bowel. Diagnosis is by laparoscopy and the treatment, which has around a 60% long term success rate, is surgical
- **polycystic ovary syndrome** (PCOS): see below. High levels of unopposed oestrogens have been implicated in chronic pelvic pain
- **residual ovary syndrome** after hysterectomy may be the result of adhesions or tethering. A recent study found that GnRH ovarian suppression was a useful test to identify an ovarian cause of post-hysterectomy chronic pain. Prolapse of the residual ovary over the vaginal vault can cause dyspareunia
- **uterovaginal prolapse** characteristically causes a dull aching pain

Non-gynaecological causes of chronic pelvic pain

- *gastrointestinal disorders* include constipation, irritable and inflammatory bowel disease, diverticular disease and malignancy
- *musculoskeletal causes* of referred pain in the lower abdomen include thoraco-lumbar disorders and hip disease
- *psychological disorder*: it is not clear whether chronic pain causes psychological disorder or whether psychological problems cause the pain. Women with chronic pelvic pain are more likely to have neurotic personalities, exhibit abnormal social attitudes and be involved in poorer quality relationships
- *renal/urinary tract causes* range from urinary tract infection, interstitial cystitis to calculi and malignancy

Treatment of chronic pelvic pain

Treatment of chronic pelvic pain, as with chronic vulval conditions, requires the health professional to take the woman's complaints and concerns seriously. This requires sympathetic, interested listening and appropriate investigation. There can be therapeutic gains from a well conducted history examination and plan of investigation. Of course, over-investigation can strengthen delusional or phobic ideas.

The differential diagnostic checklist can focus enquiries. If the problem persists without a credible diagnosis a gynaecological referral is recommended. Frequently, reassurance that no overt pathology (especially malignancy) is evident is all that is required. Laparoscopy is the investigation of choice in appropriate cases.

The principal treatment for 'essential' chronic pelvic pain and PPS is high dose progestogen therapy (medroxyprogesterone acetate 50mg/day for four months has been used). Suppression of ovulation with the combined pill is also useful. Non-specific surgical therapies include bipolar diathermy of the uterosacral ligaments (which contain abundant nerve fibres) for central pelvic pain, and pre-sacral neurectomy. Relapse after treatment is lower in women who have received psychotherapy.

Polycystic ovary syndrome

The endocrinology of PCOS is bewilderingly complex, and the family of disorders that constitute the syndrome are still being elucidated. There are, however, straightforward clinical entities where the primary care professional can offer assistance. Diagnosis is achieved using a combination of gonadotrophin level measurements (LH and FSH) and ultrasound scanning of ovarian morphology. Recent research has established links between PCOS and insulin resistance. Indeed, metformin has been used with success in affected women. For an excellent review of PCO and the metabolic syndrome see 'Polycystic ovary syndrome: metalic syndrome comes to gynaecology', *Br Med J* (1998) **317**: 329–32.

Diagnostic features

general information

General information on menarche, menstrual and fertility history are important clues in considering this diagnosis. Anovulation is a principal characteristic of PCOS. It is the consequence of a variety of endocrinological anomalies and allows ovarian oestrogen production to proceed unopposed by progesterone. The commonest cause is a high continuous secretion of LH by the pituitary. LH should be released as a mid-cycle pulse and be present at very low levels at other times. A LH/FSH level ratio >2.5 at a time other than around ovulation is suggestive of PCOS. Progesterone, the luteal phase hormone, is secreted by the corpus luteum which only develops after ovulation. Anovulation produces infertility as well as infrequent, erratic, heavy and typically painless periods: metropathia haemorrhagica. Body weight is important. Some overweight women's cycles will return to normal if they reduce their weight to normal levels. Current BMI (kg/m^2) and previous weight should be noted. Examination, looking for signs of defeminisation, androgen excess and virilisation is important in the exclusion of rare androgen-secreting tumours and in the work up of adrenal disorder. Check BP which may also be raised in adrenal conditions. Abdominal and pelvic examination may reveal enlarged ovaries. Ultrasound scanning (especially transvaginal) can show the 'pearl necklace' ovarian cysts. Refer if adrenal disease suspected. Refer if symptoms and signs are of rapid onset or if virilisation has occurred.

androgenic features

The classic features of the disorder (overweight, hirsute, oligomenorrhoeic women with acne) were described by Stein and Leventhal in the 1930s. However, many women with PCOS will not show this morphology. Those who do, respond very well to weight reduction. Hirsutism and acne can be treated as outlined in 'Hirsutism'. Anything other than mild androgenic features should prompt referral to a gynaecologist or endocrinologist: missing rare virilising tumours is the scenario to avoid. It will be useful to perform certain blood tests before your patient is seen by an endocrinologist. As mentioned earlier the pituitary gonadotrophins (FSH, LH) will be required. Serum testosterone should be measured as should Sex Hormone Binding Globulin (SHBG). If this is low it allows more testosterone to remain unbound and metabolically active. A high 17-hydroxyprogesterone level suggests adrenal 21 hydroxylase deficiency, another cause of hirsutism.

infertility

Infertility due to anovulation caused by the persistently raised level of LH is common. The miscarriage rate is also said to be higher. Ovulation induction, either with anti-oestrogens (eg. clomiphene) or gonadotrophins, has a high success rate. Ovarian diathermy, which can cause severe peri-ovarian adhesions, has been replaced by laparoscopic laser drilling or needle diathermy of the ovary as a physical treatment that can induce ovulatory cycles. Measure FSH (normal), LH (raised consistently and inappropriately; LH should surge briefly just once per cycle two weeks before menstruation), oestradiol (normal) and progesterone (absent even in the seven days before menstruation).

oligo-amenorrhoea

Oligo-amenorrhoea is caused by the tonic rather than pulsatile release of LH. Ovarian oestrogen production is satisfactory but, because of anovulation, progesterone is not produced. This causes infertility and metropathia haemorrhagica.

Clinical questions

chronic unopposed oestrogen secretion

Chronic unopposed oestrogen secretion is associated with an increased risk of endometrial cancer. For this reason, women with PCOS should take a progestogen to 'balance' the endogenous oestrogen. This applies to all PCOS women regardless of body habitus or their fertility requirements. Progestogens can be given cyclically (see under Menorrhagia) or perhaps more conveniently in the form of the combined oral contraceptive pill. The levonorgestrel intrauterine system (LNG-IUS, Mirena) would appear to be a particularly appropriate method for giving a progestogen.

hirsutism

See above.

hyperinsulinism

Hyperinsulinism is a cardiovascular risk factor and is a feature of PCOS associated with obesity. The mechanisms are still being elucidated. Weight loss appears to be an effective intervention. Research on the place of oral hypoglycaemic agents is ongoing.

infertility

Tonic LH secretion inhibits ovulation. It usually responds nicely to treatment with clomiphene. There are suggestions that if the LH level is persistently higher than 10iu/l, gonadotrophin induction and hCG support reduce the miscarriage rate. See *Chapter 5* for data on ovulation induction in primary care.

Premenstrual syndrome

PMS or the 'late luteal dysphoric syndrome' must be distinguished from the natural ebb and flow of mood that occurs from day to day and particularly in women through the menstrual cycle. The term PMS should be reserved for cases where significant symptoms exist which interfere with daily living activities. Symptom charting is required to obtain a sound diagnosis and to monitor therapeutic interventions. If symptom charts are not employed a valuable and enlightening opportunity will be missed. The term 'premenstrual dysphoric disorder' has recently been used to describe a severe form of PMS. PMDD is probably one end of the symptom spectrum of mood and mental functioning features that affect so many women. Recent work has shown that this condition responds very effectively to fluoxetine therapy.

Symptoms

PMS is a disorder of multiple symptoms, confined to the luteal phase in ovulatory women. Charting diaries are needed to list the particular symptom complexes that the individual is experiencing. These include effects on:

- *mood*: irritability, tearfulness, depression, hostility
- *cognitive function*: poor concentration, forgetfulness, confusion

- **somatic manifestations**: bloating, mastalgia, appetite disturbance, sleep disturbance, headache, tiredness
- **behaviour change**: social withdrawal, arguments

symptom charting

Symptom charting will reveal one of five patterns of distress:

- **PMS:** beginning at or shortly after ovulation and finishing at or just after the onset of menstruation. Symptoms need not be uniform throughout the luteal phase
- **Cyclic recurrence** of another disorder for example headaches, migraine, even seizures. Dysmenorrhoea is an example too
- **PMS plus another disorder:** in chronic disorder PMS symptoms may be superimposed although the chronic symptoms would not be confined to the luteal phase
- **Cyclic exacerbation** of another disorder. It is not surprising that a chronic disorder may be less bearable at a time of reduced emotional resistance. Charting would reveal its consistent presence throughout the cycle but may show it to be worse pre-menstrually
- **Non-cyclic disorder** is revealed nicely in charting diaries.

Therapy

Therapy for women with PMS begins at the first presentation with symptoms. Taking complaints seriously is vital. There may be some reluctance to take time to complete two cycles of symptom charts, but this must be encouraged as it is a therapeutic as well as a diagnostic exercise. Gaining insight into, and taking control of, her own bodily experiences may be all that some women will need (empowering). Symptom charts empower the attendant too by enabling precision in diagnosis and enabling the exact problem to be defined.

The list of therapies that have been employed in PMS is impressive. Some, like caffeine avoidance, contrast with earlier ideas of caffeine supplementation. As ever, a galaxy of therapies implies either a constellation of aetiologies or the impotence of any one intervention.

Placebos seem to be modestly effective in PMS, implying that the interest of another person and the empowerment of doing something (anything) about the problem are of themselves therapeutic. The three main interventions are: to use medications which have a central effect, to suppress ovulation and to develop strategies to tackle coexisting problems, eg. stress, relationships.

charts/symptom diaries

These are more than just a diagnostic tool as they enable women suffering with symptoms to address them directly, which can be empowering. They are also critical in making a precise diagnosis and monitoring the effect of interventions. Charts can be drawn by the patient or her attendant. They can also be purchased from the publishers of the *Drug and Therapeutics Bulletin*.

progestogens

Progestogens, in controlled trials, have never been shown to produce significant benefit. There is no progesterone deficiency in women with PMS. Indeed, progestogen therapy can evoke side-effects similar to PMS.

oestrogens

Oestrogens in the form of implants, or more recently when applied transdermally in patch form, have produced measurable benefits. Doses as low as 25mcg may be helpful. High dose unopposed oestrogen patch therapy requires the prescriber to ensure that endometrial hyperplasia is not induced. Regular endometrial biopsy is required.

antidepressants

Antidepressants have been used with some benefit. The selective serotonin re-uptake inhibitors appear to be especially beneficial in some women (eg. fluoxetine). PMDD, the more severe form of PMS which presents with mood behavioural features, responds specifically to SSRIs. Fluoxetine was licensed for this indication specifically in 1999. It is not clear whether they are treating a subliminal depressive disorder which is being unmasked only in the luteal phase by hormonal changes, or whether they have another effect. Certainly, they can be useful even in women who do not appear 'depressed'. Benzodiazepines have been found to be helpful, but the risk of dependence usually outweighs the benefit.

ovulation suppression

Ovulation suppression with the combined oral contraceptive pill has been successful. Technically women on the pill do not menstruate, they have withdrawal bleeds, and with monophasic pills there is no change in hormones from day to day. In fact, some women on the pill find the pill-free interval to be problematic because of a drop in oestrogen levels. Ovulation may also be suppressed with depot progestogens (Depo Provera and Noristerat). Danazol at 100–200 mg/day is effective but because of its side-effect potential is not a first line therapy. GnRH analogues also suppress ovulation but, in addition to their vast expense their side-effects preclude long term use.

minerals

Calcium and magnesium supplements have produced benefit in some women. Claims have also been made for zinc and copper supplements.

vitamins

Vitamins in the form of pyridoxine (vitamin B_6) are no more effective than placebos. High dose and prolonged treatment with pyridoxine can cause neurological abnormalities. Sustained treatment with doses above 200 mg/day are dangerous. Even doses as low as 50 mg/day have caused peripheral neuropathy in rare instances.

dietary modification

Some women report that caffeine withdrawal is beneficial. Others have found that increasing the carbohydrate content of the diet and reducing sugar and alcohol, as well as taking smaller but more frequent meals, is beneficial. There is no evidence that fluid and salt restriction is of benefit. An evening meal which is carbohydrate rich and protein poor has been recommended. This could have effects on serotonin metabolism.

circadian modification

Curiously, circadian modification has been shown to reduce the severity of PMS symptoms. The manoeuvre involves sleep deprivation for one night early in the luteal phase (just after ovulation). The postulated mechanism involves melitonin secretion. PMS appears to be a disorder with seasonal variations; it is frequently less troublesome in summer.

exercise

Exercise is said to reduce stress which can exacerbate other symptoms like those of PMS. There may also be an effect on endorphin metabolism in the luteal phase.

others

NSAIDs have been tried. Mefenamic acid 250 mg tds beginning 12 days before menstruation is expected, rising to 500 mg tds 9 days before and continuing this dose until the third day of the next cycle. Diuretics are to be avoided unless there is objective evidence of weight gain (5 lb in the luteal phase). Spironolactone appears to be the diuretic of choice.

placebos

Placebos appear to produce benefit in around 1:5 women. Choose an innocuous placebo.

References

Johnson SR (1992) Clinician's approach to the diagnosis and management of pre-menstrual syndrome. *Clin Obstet Gynaecol* **35**: 637–57

Anonymous (1992) Pre-menstrual syndrome. *Drug Therapeut Bull* **18**: 69–72

Prolactinoma

Prolactinoma can present gynaecologically with inappropriate lactation (galactorrhoea) and oligoamenorrhoea. It is wise to check prolactin levels in such women and in women with involuntary infertility. Laboratory ranges for prolactin vary. Prolactin is a stress hormone and an equivocal result should prompt repetition of the test. If a definite raised level is found referral to an endocrinologist is mandatory. There is no point in performing a lateral skull X-Ray examination. Just refer women with hyperprolactinaemia to a specialist after exclusion of pregnancy.

Prolapse

Prolapse means herniation of the genital tract structure(s). This can involve the vaginal walls, vaginal vault, uterus or any of these in combination. The following terms are used:

- **urethrocele**: bulging of the lower anterior vaginal wall overlying the urethra

- **urethral caruncle** is prolapse of the distal posterior urethral wall. If symptomatic (dysuria, pain, bleeding) it can be excised or cauterised

- **cystocele**: bulging of the mid and upper anterior vaginal wall overlying the urinary bladder. May be associated with discomfort and urinary control symptoms. Symptoms may respond to a well fitted vaginal ring pessary. Surgical treatment by colporrhaphy or colposuspension may be curative

- **rectocele**: bulging of the posterior vaginal wall overlying the lower rectum and anal canal. May cause discomfort and some difficulty with defecation. Responds well to surgical correction by colporrhaphy. Often associated with perineal weakness

- **enterocele**: bulging of the vaginal vault behind the cervix in the posterior fornix. The underlying relationships are the Pouch of Douglas and the general abdominal cavity. May cause discomfort. Is surgically correctable at the time of vaginal hysterectomy

- **perineal deficiency**: often the consequence of childbirth. The transverse perineal muscles are deficient and allow bulging of the anal canal into the lower vagina and fourchette. May cause discomfort and usually associated with rectocele. Surgically correctable by perinorrhaphy

- **cervical descent** implies uterine prolapse. This is the consequence of weakening of the transverse cervical ligaments, usually some years following childbirth. The definitive treatment is vaginal hysterectomy. Vaginal ring pessaries may contain the problem and are useful in the elderly, the surgically unfit or the unwilling. Symptoms include discomfort, back pain and difficulties with the use of tampons and with intercourse

- **procidentia** describes massive utero-vaginal prolapse. The vagina everts externally as the cervix and uterus descend. The cervical os may be visible at the tip of the prolapsing mass. The process drags the ureters down and may lead to hydronephrosis and renal compromise. Ulceration of the protruding mass is common. Ring pessaries may help but if the perineum is very deficient (and it usually is) they will not stay in. Packing the vagina in with dienoestrol impregnated dressings may help but beware of leaving material behind when the pack is removed. Consult a gynaecologist

Psychosexual problems

Sexuality is a central facet of human experience. Its frustrations within a relationship can be disastrous. It should be valued by the health professional. Good responses to intervention with instruction in sexual technique and psychosexual and general relationship counselling can be very rewarding. This is usually provided by experts in the field and most generalists would refer people, and hopefully couples, on. Those with a particular interest and aptitude may offer such services within primary care. It is essential that those who do take on such work are sensitive and aware of the scale of the problem: of the misery, the shattering of relationships that sexual difficulties can cause. A sensitivity for the mode of presentation is also crucial. The attendant must always be sensitive to those who may have been damaged by previous emotional or physical abuse.

Male impotence and premature ejaculation are not discussed here.

Presentation

Most individuals presenting with a sexual difficulty will probably test the waters with a non-specific somatic problem initially. Inappropriate prescriptions of antidepressants and tranquillisers and referral for gynaecological opinions is common. With sympathy, empathy and understanding problems can be revealed. The commonest cause of problems is likely to be a personal or communication difficulty within the relationship itself.

The commonest symptom complexes are:

- *aberrations of sexual expression* which are legion and cause particular difficulty if they evoke abhorrence in the partner
- *dyspareunia* may be subdivided into superficial and deep. Another classification involves

division into two categories: **intrapersonal** (due to fear, guilt, previous experiences, vaginal infection, vulval and vestibular tenderness for example) and **interpersonal** (due to relationship problems and poor communication)

- *loss of libido*, ie. impairment of desire or arousal can be the result of boredom, communication difficulties, ignorance, lack of experience, social, religious and cultural value conflict, fear of pregnancy, lack of privacy and aversion to a partner's desires
- *orgasm failure* shares many of the same factors. If sex becomes routine, is hurried, if it neglects sharing and communication aspects, concentrating only on personal genital gratification then orgasm is unlikely to be dependable
- *vaginismus* involves the involuntary contraction of pelvic floor muscles and can be a manifestation of fear of penetration

Therapy

Therapy requires taking a good social, sexual, cultural, family and relationship history. Exploring the modes of communication within the relationship is central.

- *communication*: the importance of communication circuits (sender's message, receiver's perception, receiver's feedback and the original sender's perception) should be explored and hopefully, this will lead to modification in communication habits
- *instruction* on sexual technique
- *sensate focus* was introduced by Masters and Johnson in the 1970s. By removing performance pressure (penetrative sexual intercourse) this form of behavioural therapy enables couples to embark on a voyage of self-discovery and 'pleasuring' each other. Initial sessions require time and privacy and involve a ban on the touching of breasts and genital areas. Couples take turns in giving and receiving pleasure by touching. Negative feedback is as important as positive feedback. Negative feedback is not rejection. After one or two hour-long sessions, which one commentator describes as 'homework in couple therapy', genital and breast sensate focus can be commenced, but again with a ban on penetrative intercourse. Sensate focus is particularly effective with arousal and orgasmic problems, superficial dyspareunia and vaginismus
- *couple counselling*: one commentator advised termination of counselling if no progress was being made and to offer no more than five sessions of 45–75 minutes. Endless counselling leads to a 'generally negative reaction' and provokes a 'resistance to change' (Wren B, 1985)

Wren expects a 50% short term response rate to therapy, but only a 30% response rate long term.

Reference

Wren B (1985) Psychosexual Counselling. In: Studd J, ed. *Progress in Obstetrics and Gynaecology*, vol 5: Churchill Livingstone, Edinburgh

Screening in gynaecology

General principles

One of the main tenants of medicine is *primum non nocere*: above all, do no harm. In the mind of the general public all screening must be good. However, all screens have false positive results which may lead to dangerous interventions, and false negative results which inappropriately reassure. There is even heated debate on the balance of benefits, costs, and harm done by the well established cervical cytology and mammography screening programmes. The next paragraph is written with the increasing demand for ovarian cancer and BRCA gene screening very much in mind.

Before offering a screening test (whether it be a cervical smear test, an antenatal Down's test or an over-75-years health check) ask yourself the following questions:

- have you precisely determined what it is you wish to screen for?
- is the condition being screened for a cause of significant health problems?
- does the test identify the condition earlier than it would generally present?
- does early treatment give added benefit?
- is there a suitable test?
- is the test one that people will accept?
- can you or the secondary care services cope with abnormal results?
- how often should the screening test be offered?
- what physical and emotional harm will be done to the false positives and their family/friends/fetuses?
- will the expected benefits outweigh the harm caused?
- how does the cost of screening compare with the hoped for benefits?

Types of screening

cervical intraepithelial neoplasia and cancer

Screening for CIN in order to prevent the development of invasive cancer is well established. Currently cervical cytology is the preferred method although analysing cervical epithelial cells for the presence of HPV DNA is being investigated as a free-standing screen or as an adjunct to cervical cytology. Colposcopy is too labour intensive to be offered as a first line screen, although trials have been done in primary care of cervical photography (cervicography) where the pictures are forwarded to be read by an expert.

- **brush or stick**: the purpose of cytological screening is to recover cells from the transformation zone. This may extend up the cervical canal. It has been suggested that the finding of endocervical cells on the slide indicates that an adequate smear has been taken. This theory has never been proved; indeed, one expert reviewing this question concluded that the hand that wields the spatula is of more importance than the spatula itself. If there appears to be some inflammation or friability of the cervix, especially in postmenopausal women with atrophic tissues, the use of the more gentle brush may improve the chances of obtaining an adequate sample. If bleeding is provoked the slide will be obscured by erythrocytes and will be reported as inadequate for analysis
- **hysterectomy**: most hysterectomies are 'total', that is they include removal of the cervix as well as the corpus uteri. In some cases however the cervix may not be removed, for example in the Manchester repair for prolapse, in technically difficult hysterectomies and sometimes because the surgeon or patient wishes the cervix to be preserved. Some evidence suggests that cervical conservation reduces complications and interferes less with sexual function than complete hysterectomy. In cases where hysterectomy has been performed in the presence of or because of CIN, vaginal vault cytology is advisable annually for some years

after the operation. The guidance of a gynaecologist in individual cases should be sought

- ***screen frequency:*** cervical screening should be offered every three years to women between the ages of 20–65. One study found no new cases of CIN in women over 50 years who had three negative results in the previous decade. The counsel of perfection when taking a woman's first ever smear is to take the second sample one year rather than three years later. This reduces the hazard of 'interval cancer' developing if the first smear turns out to be a false negative. There is little point in screening with cervical cytology more frequently than three-yearly intervals. This increases screening costs and the false positive rate (knock-on effect on incidence of colposcopy, biopsy, anxiety etc) with virtually no increase in the number of cases of cancer prevented

- ***screen offer***: cervical screening should be offered to all women with a cervix regardless of current or previous sexual experience. Cancer does occur in virgins

endometrial histology screening

Endometrial histology screening can be assessed in the primary care setting using one of the several varieties of biopsy devices. Most involve applying suction using a syringe attached to a catheter that is passed transcervically into the uterus. By repeatedly retracting while maintaining suction, strips of endometrium can be aspirated. Some have retractable flanges that scythe samples off. Some gynaecologists advise endometrial assessment before commencing hormone replacement therapy. There are no other routine endometrial screening indications in primary care.

osteoporosis risk screening

Osteoporosis risk screening is flavour of the month at present. There are two clinical and one pragmatic situation where this may be considered currently:

- ***to aid prophylactic therapy decision-making***: future osteopaenia risk can be quantified and tracked. If a woman is taking (or intends to take) HRT then there is no point in performing expensive screening tests simply to tell her to do what she is already doing or going to do. The gold standard test is bone densitometry and it is indicated particularly in women who would only consider 'long term' HRT if they were found to be at increased risk

- ***because of the existence of particular added risk factors*** for osteoporosis. These include:
  - premature menopause (natural or surgical)
  - steroid use
  - the other risk factors that are usually quoted for osteoporosis (ie. family history, Northern European ancestry, cigarette smoking, lack of exercise, low BMI) are poor predictors of risk. If women at increased risk are identified then bone densitometry has a place if there is a possibility that an intervention like HRT, biphosphinates or SERMs are appropriate and might be accepted by the patient

- ***patient demand*** in the increasingly litigious world of ours is a difficult one to resist. However an understanding of the principles of screening and the development of defensible guidelines can enable unreasonable demands to be resisted in good faith. Osteoporosis has a multifactorial aetiology and is amenable to a variety of therapeutic interventions. Maintaining agility into old age, regular impact exercise and sufficient calcium in the diet are easy and effective treatments. Osteoporosis is not actually the problem, fracture is the problem; so don't fall over.

ovarian cancer screening

Ovarian cancer screening is being developed. The aim will be to identify asymptomatic women with early stage and potentially curable cancer. Three tests are being assessed:

- **bimanual pelvic examination** is currently performed on women at three-year intervals when they present for cervical cytological screening. Ovarian palpation should be a part of all such examinations as the occasional stage I cancer will be detected. The ovaries shrink after the menopause and palpable ovaries should prompt further investigation, especially if the menopause was more than five years previously. The sensitivity and specificity of vaginal examination as a test for early detection of ovarian cancer is not known

- **ultrasonic scanning** can identify early tumours. However, if performed transvaginally (the preferred method) it is an invasive test. The cost per early cancer detected is huge even if restricted to women with a positive family history and therefore at higher risk. The detrimental effects of false positive results which may lead to laparoscopy etc. has to be considered

- **serum tumour marker assay** is easy and non-invasive. The antigen, CA 125, shows most promise. No national guidelines have been produced. False positives occur especially in the premenopausal, at certain times in the menstrual cycle and if endometriosis is present. A cut-off level of 30 u is usually chosen. At present most gynaecologists restrict this screen, offering it to women with a positive family history, who are already offered annual bimanual examination

There is, however, no current evidence that routine screening is of benefit. Screening women at increased risk of ovarian cancer because of a strong family history with two or more first degree relatives affected may be of benefit. The end point would be the detection of stage I (curable) ovarian cancer. Screens that detect stages III–IV ovarian disease are of little value. Women at high risk of ovarian cancer may be screened with serum marker assay and transvaginal ultrasonography annually.

vulval disease screening

Vulval disease screening is one area where the primary care professional can make a difference to a patient's life. Many vulval disorders have a pre-malignant potential. The long term sufferer or those with particular risk factors can be screened with vulval examinations annually. If doubts are raised skin biopsy or referral are the options.

Toxic shock syndrome

Toxic shock syndrome hit the headlines in the 1980s, especially in the United States. The majority of victims were found to develop the problem during menstruation and almost all used tampons. A link was established between the syndrome and the use of high absorbency fillers in certain brands of tampons. The cause of the syndrome however was liberation of *staphylococcal* toxins into the circulation. Group A *β haemolytic streptococci* have also been implicated. Since medical and public awareness has increased, and more importantly, since offending brands of tampon (that presumably allowed *staphylococci* to multiply) have been removed from the market, the incidence of the syndrome has dropped. Features of the syndrome include:

- abrupt onset of high fever
- myalgia

- diffuse skin rash with blanching erythema
- oedema
- occasionally diarrhoea and vomiting
- occasionally hypotension
- palm and sole desquamation after recovery.

Trophoblastic disease

Gestational trophoblastic disease complicates around 1:2000 pregnancies in this country. The incidence is greater in South-East Asia, with Indonesia having the highest incidence in the world at 1:85. This racial variation is reflected in the United States with Cook County reporting a rate of 1:1724 and Hawaii reporting a rate of 1:238. Trophoblast is naturally invasive but the process normally stops after placentation is complete. Even so, trophoblast can be found in the lungs of women during normal pregnancy.

Terminology

partial hydatidiform mole

This describes a focal molar change in conjunction with a live pregnancy. The maternal prognosis is better than with a complete mole as the risk of malignant transformation is lower. Pathological features of atypia are less pronounced in partial mole. The karyotype of partial molar tissue is usually triploidy XXX or XXY.

complete hydatidiform mole

Complete hydatidiform mole is the classic molar pregnancy. The karyotype is usually 46XX with both sex chromosomes being paternally derived. The risk of malignancy or malignant transformation is around 10%.

hydroptic degeneration

Hydroptic degeneration in an abortion can result in the formation of vesicles that may resemble those seen in a hydatidiform mole. Histological analysis provides the diagnosis which is important as hydroptic degeneration has no implications other than those attending an uncomplicated miscarriage.

invasive mole

Choriocarcinoma can exist in a non-metastatic form and is then known as an invasive mole which is treated in the same way as the metastatic form.

choriocarcinoma

Choriocarcinoma (chorion-epithelioma) is a malignant placental tumour. The incidence varies between 1:10000–70000 in the West and between 1:250–6000 in the Far East. Over half will follow a complete hydatidiform mole. The remainder follow spontaneous abortions, ectopic pregnancies or normal pregnancies. The maternal and paternal blood groups are related to the incidence of the disease and the prognosis: incidence being highest in couples where both are group A, lowest if both are group O, and the poorest prognostic blood group being B. The reason for this is unknown.

Clinical features

hydatidiform mole

Hydatidiform mole presents late in the first/second trimester with excessive features of pregnancy, namely rapid uterine enlargement which may cause pain, hyperemesis, theca-lutein cysts and early onset pre-eclampsia. Vesicles may be passed vaginally and there may be bleeding. Ultrasonic examination usually clinches the diagnosis with a snowstorm appearance and the absence of a fetal pole.

choriocarcinoma

Choriocarcinoma and benign trophoblastic disease tissues secrete hCG which promotes amenorrhoea. After pregnancy amenorrhoea may initially be attributed to the recent gestation or lactation. However, there will usually be associated vaginal bleeding. A positive urinary hCG test (pregnancy test) following pregnancy (aborted, ectopic or term) should prompt urgent investigation for trophoblastic disease. Choriocarcinoma may present with metastatic disease, the classic symptom being dyspnoe due to pulmonary metastases.

Management

Management is supervised by gynaecologists and oncologists. The RCOG maintains a register of all cases of trophoblastic disease in the UK and their progress is followed by one of the three supra-regional Trophoblastic Disease Reference Laboratories. The principal investigation is urinary hCG. This is tracked by the reference laboratories who send registered patients sample bottles for return. In cases of hydatidiform mole the hCG level usually falls rapidly and becomes undetectable after some weeks or months. Women with invasive mole or choriocarcinoma are also tracked with hCG levels but will invariably be offered cytotoxic therapy. Cure rates are very good. After choriocarcinoma, hCG surveillance should be continued for life.

further pregnancies

Further pregnancies should be deferred for at least six months after hCG returns to normal following hydatidiform mole and 12 months after choriocarcinoma. Surveillance is complicated by the natural rise in hCG in pregnancy. After subsequent pregnancies hCG surveillance should be re-instituted to ensure that the normal drop to unrecordable levels occurs. The risk in the UK of a second hydatidiform mole in a subsequent pregnancy is around 1:120.

oral contraception

The combined pill should not be given to women until their hCG levels have dropped to unrecordable levels.

Urinary incontinence

Urinary incontinence in women is extremely common. Rates of two or more episodes of incontinence per month occurring in half of 35-year-old women are quoted and the incidence in the elderly is considerably higher.

Causes of incontinence:

Genuine stress and detrusor instability account for 90% of cases of urinary incontinence in women.

genuine stress incontinence

This results from a mechanical inability of the mechanisms of continence to contain the normal intravesical pressure. This varies directly with intra-abdominal pressure and so coughing or straining may overwhelm the 'valves' of the bladder and urethra. Childbirth and the menopause are two physiological causes, but recurrent urinary tract infection is said to be a cause as are conditions that raise intra-abdominal pressure.

detrusor instability

Detrusor instability or bladder hyperreflexia produces incontinence because of excessive bladder contraction. The inappropriate signals cause urgency and frequency with small volume voids in addition to incontinence. The bladder in this circumstance has forgotten that it should be a reservoir as well as an expelling organ.

mixed stress and instability

Mixed stress and instability combines both the above and is diagnosed cystometrically.

retention with overflow

Retention with overflow can be caused by neurological conditions, obstructive lesions of the urethra, abdominal masses, eg. uterine fibroids and detrusor atony. It may also complicate hypothyroidism, diabetes mellitus, psychotic illness and anxiety neurosis.

functional problems

Functional problems can be complicated by incontinence resulting in either detrusor over- or under-activity.

small print causes

These include congenital anomaly, urethral diverticulae, fistulae and factitious incontinence.

Diagnosis of the cause of incontinence

At the primary care level, diagnosis of the cause of incontinence is difficult. A detailed history and examination is unreliable in distinguishing genuine stress and detrusor problems. Indeed, the term 'stress incontinence' is descriptive of a symptom and not a diagnostic entity; hence the term 'genuine stress incontinence' which can only be made on cystometric investigation. At the primary care level it is prudent to submit urine for bacteriological analysis and perhaps institute an intake and output diary incorporating times of imbibing and voiding and the volumes voided. Cystometry is the investigation of choice and is usually diagnostic.

Treatment of incontinence

This will be dependent on the diagnosis of cause.

genuine stress incontinence

This responds well to mechanical therapies. Vaginal tampons and ring pessaries may help but the definitive approaches are surgical. Anterior colporrhaphy is a poor operation unless significant cystourethrocele is present. The best operations are colposuspensions (vaginal or abdominal) and sling procedures. Collagen injections alongside the urethra are also useful in good hands. Gynaecological urology is now considered a sub-speciality and referral to a specialist with a particular interest in the subject is recommended.

detrusor irritability

Detrusor irritability often responds to simple bladder retraining (drill). This involves charting intake and, more importantly, the timing and volumes of urine output. Once a baseline is established the patient is strongly encouraged to increase the interval between voids. Relapse is not uncommon however. Some women respond to being encouraged to drink a large amount of fluid in a short time once a day. The 'cystodistension' that results can remind the bladder to act as a reservoir. Anticholinergic drugs (eg. oxybutinin) are useful. Some postmenopausal women respond well to systemic or intravaginal oestrogens. Desmopressin may be used with success for temporary relief in certain situations. Other treatments include cystodistension under anaesthesia and in severe cases bladder denervation or even diversion may be considered.

treatment

Treatment of other causes of incontinence will depend on the diagnosis, eg. diabetes or fibroids.

Vaginal discharge

Table 1.9: Vaginal discharge

	malodour*	irritation	blood stained	notes
physiological	no	no	no	Cervical and vaginal secretions are normal and vary in quality and volume with the menstrual cycle (see *chapter 3* section on natural family planning). Normality does not necessarily equate with personal preference and satisfaction
threadworms	no	yes	sometimes	An occasional cause of irritation and discharge in girls
foreign body	yes	usually	sometimes	Retained tampons can cause an overpowering and extremely distressing malodorous discharge which may be bloodstained. Foreign bodies are one of the commoner causes of discharge in young girls
candida	musty	yes	sometimes	Very common, causes vaginitis and typically with a white discharge which can be thick and curdy
bacterial vaginosis	fishy	usually not	no	A greyish discharge with fishy 'amine' odour, may be more noticeable after intercourse. No vaginitis
contraceptive pill	no	no	no	The combined pill can promote cervical ectropion. The exposed columnar epithelium produces more secretions
sexually transmitted infection	sometimes	sometimes	sometimes	A high index of suspicion must be maintained. Sexually acquired infections range from the highly symptomatic to the silent

* vaginal secretions have odour which should not be confused with malodour

Vulval disorder

In practice, generalists seeing women with vulval problems are faced with subjective symptoms and skin changes. For any one condition there can be a variety of presenting symptoms and signs which make accurate diagnosis and treatment difficult. For practical purposes, vulval disorders are presented here in a pragmatic way. There is necessarily some repetition, but this is important to achieve clarity. Vuval cancer is discussed in the 'Cancer' section above. The data is presented under four headings:

- **an overview**
- **symptoms**
- **diagnoses**
- **clinical situations**

An overview

There is a bewildering array of nomenclature on vulval pathology. However, it has been simplified recently by the International Society for the Study of Vulval Disease (ISSVD). See *Table 1.10*. Older texts may use different nomenclature but the following is the accredited terminology at present. The term 'vulval dystrophy' is no longer in vogue. Older texts may still use it alongside the terms 'hypertrophic', 'hypotrophic' and 'with or without' atypia to describe the disorders listed below. Many of these conditions are chronic in nature. Any chronic condition is attended with a pre-malignant potential. Long term follow up is therefore essential for many of these conditions.

Table 1.10: Classification of vulval skin disorder (excludes invasive cancer)

I   non-neoplastic epithelial disorders of skin and mucosa:
• Lichen sclerosis
• Squamous cell hyperplasia
• Other dermatoses
II vulval intraepithelial neoplasia (VIN)
• Squamous VIN
VIN   I mild dysplasia
VIN   II moderate dysplasia
VIN   III severe dysplasia/carcinoma in situ
• Non-squamous VIN (Paget's disease)

(Ridley *et al* (1989) *Human Pathology* **20**: 495–6)

Symptoms

There are regular complaints concerning three distinct symptom complexes. These are itching, burning and pain. In one study of British GP referrals, 70% complained of itch, 30% of burning and 10% of pain (Fischer, 1995).

- ***vulval itch*** was the most common chronic vulval symptom in Fischer's study. Pruritis is almost always accompanied by signs of excoriation and lichenification. Frequently there is erythema and occasionally oedema. In Fischer's trial over half had dermatitis, 20% had HPV and 10% had lichen sclerosus. The remainder had either VIN, psoriasis or candidiasis

- *vulval burning*, also known as vulvodynia ('pudendagra' in the USA). It is described as a chronic condition characterised by burning, stinging, irritation and a feeling of rawness. Irritation and itch appear to be different sensations. There are frequently no physical signs. Fischer's study found half of those complaining of burning had a dermatitis, the majority of the rest had HPV infection, the significance of which is not known. The remainder had lichen sclerosus, VIN, candida and dysaesthetic vulvodynia

- *vulval pain* constituted just 10% of the referrals in Fischer's study. The characteristic symptoms are entry dyspareunia and point tenderness. Vulvar vestibulitis is the classic cause

Diagnoses

Diagnosis is made as usual by taking a history and performing a complete examination in good light. Because many vulval conditions are local manifestations of generalised dermatological disorder, examination should not be confined to the vulva alone. Cytological and microbiological analysis may be appropriate. Vulval skin biopsy often enables a precise diagnosis to be achieved. It may be necessary to biopsy several sites. The technique of punch biopsy is especially suited to the vulva:

- **atrophic changes** can develop after the menopause. The vulva becomes red and inflamed on a background of skin pallor. Ulceration may occur. The condition may mimic lichen sclerosis. Topical and even systemic oestrogens can be very effective

- **bacterial vaginosis** has been linked with vulval symptomatology and is easily diagnosed. A grey, offensive discharge may be present

- **candidiasis** is an occasional cause of vulvitis. Always check for and, if necessary, treat vaginitis. Use imidazole preparations as nystatin is ineffective on the vulva

- **cervicitis** is said to be a cause of vulval symptoms. It is easily diagnosed by inspection and bacteriological testing. See above

- **dermatitis** was found by Fischer in over half of the cases referred for a secondary care opinion. Possible causes include an atopic history (although atopy generally spares the vulva), allergy and irritants. Allowing the vulva to ventilate by appropriate choice of clothing and keeping the area dry is essential. In cases of pruritis it is vital to break the itch/scratch cycle. Avoidance of irritants (especially soaps, deodorants and topical anaesthetic agents) and use of emollients is important. Topical corticosteroids in mild form for prolonged use or moderate potency for up to eight weeks use are effective

- **dysaesthetic vulvodynia**, for example, following herpetic infection. Frequently no cause is found, 'essential vulvodynia', and in such instances the cause is thought to lie in the neural pathways from the vulval skin. This can occur at the level of the nerve endings or higher up where impulses are modulated. There can also be higher perceptual problems. Antidepressants can be effective in such cases and it is thought they work on the neural pathways rather than on the psyche

- **eczema** may be part of a generalised condition or be the consequence of application of local irritants (soap, detergent, deodorisers, antihistamines, local anaesthetic preparations, perfumes, spermicides, rubber). Seborrhoeic dermatitis is discussed below

- **generalised pruritic disorder** includes diabetes, cholestasis, hepatitis, uraemia, lymphoma and iron deficiency. Treatment is aimed at the primary cause

- **HPV infection** may be found histologically in the absence of macroscopic change. The presence of condyloma accuminata should prompt referral to a genitourinary specialist. Treatment with low strength topical costicosteroids can alleviate pruritis. The relationship between microscopic HPV changes and symptoms is not known; the association may well be casual. HPV is associated with malignant change. Long term follow up is therefore essential

- **hyperplastic change** was formerly known as hyperplastic dystrophy. If atypical features (now known as VIN) are present on histological analysis of biopsy material referral to a gynaecologist is essential as there is a malignant potential. In the absence of VIN, attention to ventilation and elimination of irritants is essential. Low strength topical corticosteroid or short term (up to eight weeks) moderate strength topical corticosteroid can give useful relief. In severe cases triamcinolone injections can be tried (secondary care procedure). Annual follow up with vulval examination is recommended. Mixed changes with hyperplasia and atrophy coexisting can occur

- **intertrigo,** or inflammation in the flexures is usually caused by fungal infections, such as tinea, and usually responds to improved ventilation and the application of topical imidazoles with or without steroids

- **lichen planus** is an uncommon but important cause of vulval symptoms. There may be accompanying skin changes elsewhere and, of course, the characteristic buccal signs should be sought

- **lichen sclerosus** is the female equivalent of balanitis xerotica obliterans. The diagnosis is made histologically. The principal symptom is pruritis and the clinical features are a pale, atrophic, crinkly skin change with telangiectasia and purpura. The skin may be fissured and eventually shrinks and thins making intercourse uncomfortable or even impossible. Treatment is with potent topical steroids and emollients. Topical testosterone is often effective. There is a link between lichen sclerosus and autoimmune disease, particularly of the thyroid. One study has found that 75% of women with LS had at least one auto-antibody and 20% had an autoimmune disease. The involvement of a dermatologist is advisable. Lichen sclerosus has a pre-malignant potential

- **lichen simplex** tends to occur in younger women than lichen sclerosus. Whether it provokes or is the result of scratching is unclear. It produces a thickened red and scaly hyperkeratotic skin change. It responds to emollients and topical steroids. The itch/scratch cycle must be broken. Associated VIN/carcinoma is a real hazard

- **peri-orificial dermatitis** is a consequence of prolonged moderate or potent topical corticosteroid use. Withdrawal of steroids produces an initial flare up of symptoms but is usually followed by a good response

- **psoriasis** has a predilection for the genital area. Signs of it should be sought elsewhere including the nails. Treatment is best offered in conjunction with a dermatologist

- **psychological disorder** may present with vulval symptoms although it is generally thought that persistent vulval symptoms are more likely to be the cause of psychological problems rather than be the result of them

- **seborrhoeic dermatitis** may be accompanied by seborrhoeic signs elsewhere (particularly pre-sternal, on the face, brows, ears and in the scalp). A diffuse pink reddening of the vulval skin, especially in the crural folds, will be evident. Treat with topical steroids

- **sexually transmitted disease**, for example trichomonas, chancre, syphilis and herpes virus infection must always be considered, especially if there is ulcer ation. Refer to a GUMed specialist if in doubt
- **urinary tract infection** is said to be a cause of vulval symptoms
- **vesiculobullous diseases** are a rare cause of vulval complaint. Fixed drug eruptions should be considered and a dermatological opinion sought
- **VIN/carcinoma** *in situ*, previously known variously as dysplasia and Bowenoid papulosis, is often extensive and multifocal. It presents with reddened raised plaques. It is increasingly presenting in younger women. There is a definite link with CIN and with cigarette smoking. Paget's disease tends to be red, moist and scaly

- **vulval cancer** may present as a thickening in the vulval skin. Ulceration should always raise the possibility of malignancy. Malignant melanoma also occurs on the vulva
- **vulvar vestibulitis** presents with introital dyspareunia and point tenderness over the skin of the vestibule. It may be triggered by infections such as candidiasis. HPV infection may have a role in its aetiology. There is usually little to see on inspection other than diffuse redness. Treatments include emollients, topical steroids and local anaesthetic gels (especially prior to intercourse), however these can lead to skin sensitisation. In resistant and severe cases surgical vestibulectomy is an option

Clinical situations

- **atrophic change of the vulva**: consider postmenopausal vulval atrophy but do not omit to consider lichen sclerosus
- **cystic lesions of the vulva** are generally sebaceous if located on the hair-bearing skin and mucous if on the glabrous skin of the vestibule. The Bartholin's glands are the largest of the vestibular mucous glands. Unlike sebaceous cysts, mucous gland cysts can be caused by sexually transmitted infection. Vulval hydroceles related to the vestigial Woolfian ducts can produce cystic swellings deep into the external vulval skin
- **dermatoses of the vulva** range from irritant eczemas and seborrhoeic dermatitis through to generalised skin disorders, such as psoriasis and lichen planus. Vesiculobullous disorders can also occur on the vulva. Examination should not be limited to the vulval skin alone. Biopsy can be diagnostic
- **erythematous lesions**: these must always be taken seriously. Causes range from topical infection (eg. tinea) through

lichen sclerosus and hyperplastic change to the neoplastic disorders. Again biopsy may be diagnostic. Lichen planus tends to be violaceous
- **excoriated lesions**: scratching of the vulva may be the cause of symptoms (lichen simplex) or the result of other disorders (eg. lichen sclerosus). Breaking the itch/scratch cycle is the first priority of treatment. Again biopsy in difficult cases may be diagnostic
- **pigmented lesions of the vulva** need urgent referral as malignant melanoma is a real possibility. Most pigmented lesions will however be simple freckles.
- **pruritis vulvae** is the commonest of vulval symptoms. It can be a feature of most disorders ranging from transient infection through dermatoses to the pre-malignant disorders. Vulval cancer itself can evoke pruritis. Obviously it must always be taken seriously and, if persistent, referral and regular screening should be considered

- **ulcerated lesions of the vulva** can be caused by infection, trauma, atrophy and tumour. In most cases an appropriate referral will be indicated (to dermatologist, gynaecologist or GU Medicine specialist). Ulceration may be caused by obscure conditions like Behçet's disease or may accompany Crohn's disease

- **warty lesions of the vulva** may indeed be viral warts (condyloma accuminata). It must be remembered that syphilis can produce vulval warts (condylomata lata) and the warty change may be accompanied by, and perhaps can cause, neoplasia (either VIN or vulval cancer)

Frequently no physical cause can be found and treatments may be less than satisfactory. However, it is essential that the symptom be taken seriously. One commentator stated that the physician's attitude in trying to seek out a cause was the single most important factor in treating this disorder. Many women will be greatly reassured to know that their symptom is not the consequence of sexually transmitted disease or malignancy.

References

Fischer G (1995) The chronically symptomatic vulva: aetiology and management. *Br J Obstet Gynaecol* **102**: 773–9

Ridley CM *et al* (1989) New nomenclature for vulval diseases. *Human Pathology* **20**: 495–6

2
the change

In all countries of the world, women who live long enough will reach a stage in their lives when the hormonal function of the ovaries wanes and eventually ceases. The process occurs over a period of years and is commonly called 'the change' or climacteric. The change is not a disease but a natural transition; a part of a woman's natural development and the ageing process. It can be smooth and trouble free or it may be exceedingly uncomfortable. It comes at a time of gradually increasing cardiovascular risk and is eventually followed in some women by skeletal problems. But, more positively, it is also a time in life when a woman is free of menstruation, dysmenorrhoea, pre-menstrual symptoms and, of course, the risk of pregnancy.

This chapter looks at the climacteric. It rigidly distinguishes between symptomatic treatment of climacteric symptoms (straightforward) and the prophylactic uses of HRT to prevent disease and prolong life (a therapeutic dilemma). Specific data is listed under the principal therapeutic agent headings. Numerous tables display data that will be of use during consultation.

Chapter contents

The usual age of menopause is just over 50. Onset is hastened by:

- **cigarette smoking:** which can hasten onset of menopause by up to two years

- **altitude:** long term living at high altitude is associated with earlier menopause

- **hysterectomy:** even when ovaries are conserved, hysterectomy produces changes in pelvic vasculature that lead to earlier ovarian senescence

- **familial:** early menopause seems to run in families

- **premature ovarian failure**.

Key issues

There are three major areas to be considered when discussing the change with women:
- acceptance of the change without hormone replacement
- symptomatic treatment
- prophylactic treatment.

acceptance of the change; no hormone replacement

This almost sounds heretical but it is in fact what most women actually do. The change is of course a natural development and intervention needs justification. As discussed below, therapeutic questions relate to symptomatic treatment and prophylactic therapy. The assumption that 'there has to be a good reason not to use HRT' is debatable, and for those with few symptoms and no special risk factors it can be difficult to justify. The prospect of long term potential benefit may be outweighed by anxieties about breast cancer, the continuation of periods and the attendant medical treatment that follows.

symptomatic treatment in the change

This does not present many dilemmas to the prescriber. The issues are subjective and quality related. An assessment of contraindications to HRT has to be made but, thereafter, the decision to take or continue therapy rests mainly with the woman experiencing the symptoms. Many will choose a therapeutic trial of HRT. A review of benefits and side effects should be made two or three months later.

The principal areas where symptomatic therapy is indicated are:
- *vasomotor symptoms* (flushing, sweats, sleep disturbance)
- *psychological symptoms* (mood, concentration, memory)
- *urogenital symptoms* (urgency, dysuria, vaginal dryness).

prophylactic treatment and the change

This presents many dilemmas for the prescriber. A balance of supposed risks to be averted versus an estimate of the detrimental effects of therapy must be made with each individual woman. The published data is contradictory but a large meta-analysis by Grady (1992) provides some guidance. Grady's analysis estimated the lifetime risks of disease and the effects of therapy on healthy fifty year old white women. Further analysis looked at risks and benefits to women at increased risk of particular conditions (eg. with a family history of breast disease, pre-existing coronary artery disease). The data has to be interpreted with caution. Prescribing habits are different in North America and it is not clear how applicable the data is for other ethnic groups. For example, osteoporosis does not appear to be a problem for women of Afrocarribean origin.

Tables 2.1–3 present some of the Grady data. It can be seen that HRT appears to give protection against coronary artery disease and osteoporotic hip fracture, but the reductions in risk and prolongation of life found in this analysis are modest. The increased risk of breast cancer in users of HRT compared with non-users is also modest. *Table 2.3* presents Grady's data on the risk of disease and benefits of HRT in women identified as being at greater than average risk of bone, breast or heart disease. The issues are well discussed by Pereira Gray *et al* (1995), Davidson (1995) and Utian (1996). Almost all the published studies on the long term benefits of HRT are observational and short term, relying on surrogate markers of disease rather than the disease itself (eg. lipid changes rather than myocardial infarction). They are generally open to selection bias and the effects of the 'health cohort' phenomenon.

The key systems where prophylactic use of HRT and other therapies is of importance are:

- **skeletal** (protection against osteoporosis): There is no doubt that oestrogens stop, and may even reverse, bone demineralisation. However, only a minority of women are destined to become osteoporotic and not all of those who do will sustain a fracture. Non-oestrogen skeletal protection can be achieved by attention to diet (eg. calcium in post-menopausal women), cessation of smoking and regular weight bearing exercise. These are protective of bone mass, although calcium supplements are only of real use in the established osteoporotic. Osteoporotic hip and wrist fractures are almost exclusively seen in women who fall. Attention to the disposition of furniture and carpets, for example, can reduce the risk of falls . Regular exercise, in addition to strengthening bones, maintains proprioceptive responses which also protect against falls and so against fractures. Vertebral wedge fracturing and the kyphotic Dowager's Hump is not so amenable to prevention other than with oestrogen HRT, bisphosphinates, SERM's and to a lesser extent calcium. The lifetime risk of an osteoporotic fracture for a fifty-year-old woman is around 15%. 'Ever use' of HRT reduces it to around 12% (Grady D, 1992). See *Tables 2.1–2.3*.

- **cardiovascular** (protection against coronary artery disease): the lifetime risk of CAD for a fifty-year-old woman is around 45%. Oestrogen HRT reduces it to 34% according to Grady. But, as with the other big questions about HRT, there is controversy. Postuma (1994) contended that the bane of epidemiological surveys 'selection bias' may account for much of the perceived benefits. The consensus view is that oestrogens are a good thing for the coronary arteries. This view is supported by the nurses' health study (Stampfer MJ, 1991). The addition of a progestogen may have a detrimental effect, but the magnitude if any is small. Transdermal delivery of the oestrogen appears to be marginally less cardioprotective than the oral route. The cardioprotective effects may be greatest in women at special risk of cardiac events (eg. smokers, diabetics and those with established ischaemic heart disease). See *Tables 2.1–2.4*. However, the only prospective randomised trial reported to date assessing the relationship between HRT use and coronary artery disease failed to demonstrate benefit (Hulley S, 1998).

- **breast** (increased risk of breast cancer): the evidence of the magnitude of the risk is contradictory, but with British women having the highest incidence of breast cancer in the world the issue is crucial. The consensus is that the risk of breast cancer is increased in women who take oestrogens for five or more years. The nurses' health study found a 50% increase in breast cancer in women who took oestrogens for five or more years (Colditz, 1995). The increased risk was even greater in women using oestrogens in their sixties and seventies. As can be seen from Grady's data however, there is also a significant risk of the disease in women who do not take oestrogens. The Collaborative Group on Hormone Factors and Breast Cancer recently reported new evidence confirming a definite increase in breast cancer with HRT use but the rise, although dependent on duration of use of HRT, was very small and decreased rapidly after cessation of therapy. Also the cancers that were seen in HRT users were less advanced (Collaborative Group, 1997: see *Table 2.5*). The balance between risk and benefit where the indication for using oestrogens is symptomatic is usually not too difficult, although guidance from a breast surgeon or an oncologist may enable the woman to make a more informed decision. The use of oestrogens as prophylactic therapy in women with a larger than average breast cancer risk is very difficult especially if there are no particular features suggesting excessive skeletal or cardiovascular vulnerability. The risk factors are a family history of breast cancer, especially onset before the age of fifty in one or more first degree relatives, and a personal history of benign breast disease where there has been evidence of proliferation. See *Tables 2.1–2.3 and 2.5*.

- **venous thromboembolism** (increased risk of DVT and pulmonary embolism): The use of oestrogens whether in the combined contraceptive pill or HRT slightly increases the risk of DVT and PE. Several observational studies are in agreement that the background risk in post-menopausal women is around 10 per 100,000 women per year. Oestrogen HRT use increases it to around 30/100,000. However, the risk is highest in the first six months of use. Thrombophylia screening is not recommended in general, although the RCOG recommend that women with a personal or family history of DVT/PE should be screened and counselled on their individual risks and anticipated benefit with HRT. It is recommended that this is done by a specialist in thrombophilia. HRT need not be stopped prior to surgery but should be considered a factor enhancing the risk of DVT/PE alongside age, obesity, immobility and infection. Anti-coagulation and compression stockings should be considered in such instances. The *RCOG Guideline Number 19*, April 1999, discusses the subject with clarity and provides useful guidance, as does a recent number of the *Drug and Therapeutics Bulletin* (1999, **37**: 78–80) for those wishing to know more.

- **length and quality of life** is marginally greater in oestrogen users. Grady's figures suggested that it was not very large. Remember that there are no randomised controlled trials to give definite answers to this question. Length of life among HRT users depends on the balance of risk of breast cancer (and how quickly that risk falls after cessation of therapy) versus the benefit of cardiac protection (and how long it is maintained after HRT is terminated). Women at particular risk of breast cancer may have less to gain than women at particular risk of ischaemic heart disease. There is a good review of the issues by Nancy Davidson (Davidson N, 1995). See *Tables 2.1–2.5*.

- **Alzheimer's disease** is probably not prevented by oestrogens. However recent data suggest that the onset of the disease may be deferred significantly; in some individuals beyond the natural life span of the individual. The effects seen in one study suggested that the benefits were greater in those who took oestrogens longer. The mechanism may be a direct effect on neurones by protecting them against amyloid ß deposition and intracellular neurofibrillary tangle formation. An indirect effect on the cerebral vasculature involving vessel wall compliance is also possible. The relative risk of Alzheimer's disease in oestrogen users in one observational study was 0.4 (Tang M-X, 1996). Should a significant preventative effect be proved then the risk benefit balance of long term HRT use would move towards benefit.

Table 2.1: Future risk of disease in a white 50-year-old woman and the effect of HRT

	Lifetime risk of developing disease %	Lifetime risk of dying of the disease %	Median age at presentation (years)	Relative risk in women using HRT	
endometrial cancer	2.6	0.3	68	E+P E	RR 1.0 RR 2.3 **
breast cancer	10	3	69	E > 8 years	RR 1.25
coronary artery disease	46	31	74 *	E	RR 0.65
osteoporotic hip fracture	15	1.5	79	E (ever) E > 10 years	RR 0.75 RR 0.5

Table 2.2: Lifetime chances of disease in users and non-users of HRT

		Non use of HRT	Oestrogen use	Oestrogen + Progestogen use
CAD	%	46.1	34.2	34.4
hip fracture (osteoporotic)	%	15.3	12.7	12.8
breast cancer	%	10.2	13.0	13.0
endometrial cancer**	%	2.6	19.7	2.6
life expectancy	years	82.8	83.7	83.8

Table 2.3: Effects of HRT on future health and lifespan in women with risk factors

		Lifetime probability *	Probability in oestrogen users	Probability in oestrogen and progestogen users
women at risk of CAD	%	71.2	59.6	59.8
women at risk of osteoporotic hip fracture	%	36.2	31.4	31.6
women at risk of breast cancer#	%	19.3	24.1	24.2

(Ref. Grady, 1992)

Notes:
Assumes that progestogens will not have detrimental effects
E   oestrogen
P   progestogen
CAD coronary artery disease
*   death
**   in non-hysterectomised women
#   risk defined as mother or sister with breast cancer

Table 2.4: Effects of various HRT formulations on serum lipids

	Oral oestrogen	Transdermal oestrogen	Effect of addition of an androgenic progestogen	Tibolene
TC	↓ slightly	↓	↑	↓
HDL	↑	? small ↓	↓	↓
LDL	↓	↓	↑	no data
Triglycerides	↑	small ↓	↓	↓
Atherogenic index	↓	↑	no data	↑

(Principal source: Hanggi W, 1997)

Table 2.5: Cumulative incidence of breast cancer per 1,000 current or recent HRT users

Up to age years	Never use	5 years use	10 years use	15 years use
50	18	18	18	18
55	27	28	28	28
60	38	40	41	41
65	50	52	56	57
70	63	65	69	75
75	77	79	83	89

(The Collaborative Group on Hormone Factors in Breast Cancer, 1997)

The principal therapeutic options are:

- **supportive** This may be all that some women wish or need. Discussion of the problems and symptoms they are encountering alongside the benefits of being post-menopausal (no periods, pregnancies or PMT) can be very therapeutic

- **lifestyle questions** can be addressed at a time when many women are particularly receptive. Smoking cessation, diet and exercise are particularly appropriate subjects for discussion

- **hormonal preparations** Systemic preparations are discussed further below and details of available formulations and products are listed in tables. Topical oestrogen acts on the vaginal epithelium counteracting atrophy and promoting vaginal moisture. They are helpful in cases of recurrent vaginal infection, the urethral syndrome and in some instances prior to pelvic surgery

- **SERMs, minerals and biphosphinates** Calcium supplements are helpful in post-menopausal women with established osteoporosis but are not protective against the rapid bone mineral loss around the time of the menopause. They are also given alongside biphosphinates which increase bone mass by remineralisation. Raloxifene, the first SERM, became available autumn 1998. They have an oestrogen like effect on bone, are inert on the endometrium and appear to have a protective effect on the breast.

Oestrogen therapy

Box 2.1: Oestrogen therapy data

Indications: Relief of menopausal symptoms, prophylaxis against long-term oestrogen deficiency (coronary artery disease, osteoporosis)

Cautions: Migraine, severe headaches occurring for the first time on treatment, chronic liver disease, cholelithiasis and conditions that can deteriorate in pregnancy, such as multiple sclerosis, epilepsy, diabetes mellitus, hypertension, porphyria, tetany, uterine fibroids, family history of breast cancer, congenital lipid disorders

Contraindications: Pregnancy, severe liver disease, otosclerosis that has deteriorated in pregnancy, thromboembolic disorder, sickle cell anaemia, hormone dependent disorder or tumour, eg. carcinoma of the breast

Interactions: ACE inhibitors, rifampicin, antagonism of anticoagulants, antagonism of antidepressants and increased side-effects of tricyclics, antagonism of antidiabetic drugs, anti-epileptics and barbiturates accelerate oestrogen metabolism, antagonism of hypotensive effects of anti-hypertensives, cyclosporin plasma level increased

Prescribing choices

- **continuous combined HRT** involves giving a daily dose of both oestrogen and progestogen. The dose is fixed and there are no breaks in therapy. The result is that in women with no residual ovarian activity the endometrium thins to a degree that withdrawal bleeding does not occur. Initially hailed as 'bleed free HRT' it is now more modestly advertised as 'period free HRT'. See *Table 2.8*.

- **implants** are available as 17ß oestradiol and testosterone. They have the advantage of producing a smooth and prolonged effect, lasting on average six months. They do, however, have to be implanted using a trochar set under local anaesthesia. Once the crystalline pellet is implanted it cannot be removed and so in situations where HRT is being given as a trial (especially in women with a past history of endometriosis) it would be wrong to use implants. Oestradiol implants are effective against osteoporosis and the addition of testosterone is very effective where lower libido is a problem (*Table 2.12*). Tachyphylaxis can be a problem with implants. This means that the dose required to produce a given response increases with each successive implant. Supra-physiological plasma levels may be required to give benefit ultimately. It is advised that measuring serum oestradiol level prior to each implant be done to look for this. Testosterone implants are generally used where reduced libido is a major factor.

- **natural oestrogens** are used in the change to mimic rather than to suppress the action of the ovary. Oestradiol is the principal oestrogen. Oestriol and oestrone are the two other natural human oestrogens. Although oestradiol is a constituent of many of the oral formulations, it is transformed during absorption into oestrone. The same fate awaits both oral oestriol and the conjugated equine oestrogens. Only transdermal and subcutaneous implants deliver oestradiol itself to the circulation.

- **opposed oestrogens** are ones that have a progestogen incorporated into the regime. This can be given orally, transdermally or topically using vaginal progesterone gel (intrauterine therapy with the LNG-IUS may be permissible in the future). It is usual to use opposed oestrogens in non-hysterectomised women. The 1960s American 'feminine forever' approach using unopposed oestrogens in non-hysterectomised women was followed by a massive rise in the endometrial cancer rate. If unopposed oestrogens are given to women who have not had their uterus removed then regular endometrial surveillance is essential (either by endometrial biopsy, hysteroscopy or transvaginal ultrasound scan). See *Tables 2.6–2.8*.

- **oral oestrogens** are available as oestradiol, oestrone, oestriol and conjugated oestrogens of equine origin. All are transformed during the absorption process into oestrone. The synthetic oestrogen mestranol is also used for HRT (*Tables 2.6 and 2.8*).

- **phytoestrogens** are plant derived compounds with oestrogenic activity. There are two principal groups; the lignans which include linseed and the isoflavones which are found in legumes such as soybeans. In some parts of the world a considerable proportion of the diet consists of phytoestrogen rich foods and women from these regions appear to suffer less with climacteric symptoms. Very little objective data is available on their effects in climacteric women, however, they have been shown to suppress gonadotrophin levels. More research is needed before reliable opinions can be given. Of some concern is the possibility that an unopposed oestrogenic effect on the endometrium and breast could be deleterious in the long term. Phytoestrogen products are available and are being marketed to women as an alternative to pharmacological HRT, however the data on their benefits and safety is not yet available.

- **sequential opposed oestrogens** involve the addition of ten to fourteen days of progestogen treatment per cycle. This 'balancing' of hormones reduces the risk of development of endometrial hyperplasia which can progress through atypia to endometrial carcinoma. See *Tables 2.6 and 2.7*.

- **synthetic oestrogens** are mainly used in contraceptive pills to suppress the ovary. Apart from mestranol there are no routine situations where they are used in the change apart from their use in the combined oral contraceptive pill.

- **topical oestrogens** are all for use within the vagina. All are designed for short or medium term use. Prolonged use is unusual and then only with periodic breaks in treatment to assess continuing need. Although poorly absorbed, prolonged use may cause endometrial stimulation. They are available as creams, pessaries and intravaginal medicated rings. Beware: the more potent topical oestrogens (dienoestrol, stilboestrol and Premarin) are absorbed systemically and anything more than brief exposure requires progestogen opposition in the un-hysterectomised. Absorption through the penile skin during intercourse has been known to cause male gynaecomastia. Some products can damage latex (*Table 2.10*).

- **transdermal gel oestradiol** has been popular in France for several years and was introduced into the United Kingdom in 1995. Gel is applied from a pressurised canister giving metered doses or small sachets to an area of skin on the arm, shoulders or thighs once a day. The skin of the vulva and breast should be avoided. Although applied to skin, the action of the gel is systemic not local, hence their listing under the transdermal oestrogens (*Table 2.7*).

- **transdermal patch oestrogens** all deliver 17ß oestradiol. They are applied either in patch form or as a transdermal gel. The first patches contained oestradiol in an alcoholic reservoir. The second generation patches contain oestrogen within the adhesive and are known as matrix patches. It is claimed that second generation patches cause less skin irritation and come unstuck less often than the first generation reservoir patches. The delivery of hormone is also smoother throughout the 3–4 day period. Matrix patches are thinner and more translucent making them more 'discreet'. Skin irritation is said to be less problematic if patches are applied to the buttock rather than the abdomen or back. Patches are replaced once or twice per week (*Tables 2.7 and 2.8*).

- **unopposed oestrogens** can be used safely in women who have had a hysterectomy. Their use in women with an intact uterus can lead through atypia to endometrial cancer. Regular uterine surveillance with transvaginal ultrasound, hysteroscopy or endometrial biopsy is required if this option is chosen. See *Tables 2.6–2.7 and 2.10*.

Table 2.6: HRT: Oral oestrogens

Preparation	Oestrodiol dose	Progestin dose	Osteoporosis licence	Notes *
unopposed				
Ellest solo	I mg, 2 mg		2 mg only	
Climaval	I mg, 2 mg			
Progynova	I mg, 2 mg		2 mg only	
Zumenon	I mg, 2 mg		2 mg only	
Harmogen	-		√	oestrone as estropipate
Hormonin	-		√	various oestrogens
Premarin	0.62, 1.25, 2.5 mg		√	5–10 years use required
opposed sequential				
NET combinations				
Climagest	I mg, 2 mg	I mg	2 mg only	
Ellest duet	I mg, 2 mg	I mg		
Trisequens	2/2/I mg	I mg	√	
Trisequens forte	4/4/I mg	I mg	√	
LNG/NORG combinations				
Cycloprogynova	I mg	250 mcg		
Cycloprogynova	2 mg	500 mcg	√	
Nuvelle	2 mg	75 mcg	√	
Prempak-C 0.625 and 1.25	-	*I50 mcg	√	CEO
MPA combinations				
Premique cycle	-	*I0 mg	√	CEO 0.625 mg
Tridestra	2mg	20 mg	√	Quarterly bleed
DDG combinations				
Femoston I/10	I mg	I0 mg		
Femoston 2/10	2 mg	I0 mg	√	
Femoston 2/20	2 mg	20 mg	√	

Principal source: *MIMS*, November 1999; *BNF* **38**, September 1999

Notes:

Mestranol is an inactive product which converts to ethinyloestradiol in vivo

* indicates that the progestogen is not combined with the oestrogen in a single pill but comes as a separate pill
This is important as it is known that for some women there is a temptation to omit the progesten if it causes unwanted effects

Table 2.7: HRT: Transdermal oestrogens

Product	dose/ 24hrs	Progestogen	Progestogen dose	Osteoporosis licence	Notes
unopposed					
Dermestril				-	
Estraderm TTS and MX	25 mcg			-	
Evorel				-	
Menorest	37.5 mcg			-	
Ellest solo MX	40 mcg				
Fematrix **				-	aqueous matrix
Dermestril				-	
Estraderm TTS & MX				√	
Evorel	50 mcg			√	
Femseven *				√	7 day patch
Menorest				√	
Progynova TS *				-	7 day patch
Estraderm MX					
Evorel	75mcg			√	
Femseven *				√	7 day patch
Menorest				√	
Ellest solo MX	80 mcg			√	
Fematrix **				√	aqueous matrix
Dermestril				-	
Estraderm TTS & MX				-	
Evorel	100 mcg			√	
Femseven *				√	7 day patch
Progynova TS *				-	7 day patch
Oestragel	1.5 g			√	transdermal gel
Sandrena	0.5 mg			-	transdermal gel
Sandrena	1.0 mg			-	transdermal gel
opposed					
Femapak 40 **	40 mcg	DDG	10 mg	-	patch/tabs
Evorel pak	50 mcg	NET	1 mg	√	patch/tabs
Estracombi	50 mcg	NET	250 mcg	√	res' patch
Estrapak	50 mcg	NET	1 mg	√	patch/tabs
Evorel sequi	50 mcg	NET	170 mcg	√	MX patch
Nuvelle TS	50/80 mcg	LNG	20 mcg	-	phased MS patches, 50mcg + 80mcg with LNG tablet
Femapak 80 **	80 mcg	DDG	10 mg	√	patch/tabs

Principal source: *MIMS*, November 1997

Table 2.8: HRT: 'Continuous combined' oestrogens

Product	Oestrogen dose	Progestogen	Progestogen dose	Osteoporosis licence	Notes
Climesse	2 mg	NET	0.7 mg	√	
Elleste duet conti	2 mg	NET	I mg		
Evorel Conti	50 mcg	NET	I70 mcg	√	100% TDX
Kliofem	2 mg	NET	1.0 mg	√	
Kliovance	I mg	NET	0.5 mg		
Livial	2.5 mg	-	-	√	tibolone
Nuvelle Continuous	2 mg	NET	I mg	√	
Premique	0.625 mg	MPA	5 mg	√	CEO

Principal source: *MIMS* November 1999; *BNF* **38**, September 1999

Table 2.9: HRT: Progestogens that may be used with unopposed oestrogens

Product	Progesten	Dose	Notes
Micronor HRT	NET	I mg x 36	higher dose than POP, lower than Primolut N
Duphaston HRT	DDG	10 mg x 42	
Crinone	Progesterone	4%	6 loaded applicators of vaginal gel
(Mirena)	LNG	20mcg/day	LNG-IUS; unlicensed application

Progestogen therapy

Box 2.2: Progestogen therapy data

Indications: To balance oestrogens used in hormone replacement in women who have not had a hysterectomy. Progestogens may be used as HRT for vasomotor symptoms on their own in women who cannot take oestrogens

Cautions: Diabetes mellitus, hypertension, liver disorder, lipid anomalies, prior mastopathy and family history of breast cancer, multiple sclerosis, gall stones, uterine fibroids, systemic lupus erythematosis, porphyria, asthma and melanoma

Contraindications: Severe liver disorder or history of jaundice or pruritis in pregnancy, history of pemphigoid gestations, pregnancy, acute venous thromboembolism

Interactions: Barbiturates, hydantoins, meprobramate, phenylbutazone, rifampicin, activated charcoal, cyclosporin

Prescribing choices

- **continuous combined progestogens** are given alongside oestrogens without a break every day. They do not work by promoting secretory change and endometrial shedding, but by thinning the endometrium. By avoiding hormone withdrawal they also avoid withdrawal bleeding. They cannot be used too close to the menopause as erratic bleeding is likely. Six formulations are currently available, see *Table 2.8.*

Table 2.10: HRT: Topical oestrogens

Product	Oestrogen	Pack data	Dose	Notes
Creams				
Ortho-dienoestrol*	dienoestrol	78 g	1–2 applicatorfuls/ day reduce for maintenance	potent oestrogen with systemic absorption
Ortho-gynest *	oestriol	80 g	1 applicatorful/day, reduce for maintenance	
Ovestin	oestriol	15 g	1 applicatorful/day, x 2–3 weeks, reduce for maintenance	
Premarin	CEO	42.5 g	1–2 g/day for 3 weeks followed by 1 weeks rest	0.625mg/g, potent oestrogen, systemic absorption
Vaginal tabs/pessaries				
Ortho-gynest *	oestriol	0.5 mg x 15	1 tablet/day, reduce for maintenance	
Tampovagan	stilboestrol	0.5 mg x 10	2 pv nocte for 2–3 weeks	potent oestrogen with sytemic absorption
Ovestin	oestriol	1 mg x 30	½tabs –3 tabs/day x 1 month. Reduce for maintenance	
Vagifem	oestradiol	25 mcg x 15	1 x 2 weeks then twice weekly. Reassess after 3 months	
Vaginal ring				
Estring	oestradiol	7.5 mcg/24 hours	replace three monthly, do not use longer than 2 years	

(Principal source: *MIMS*, November 1999; *BNF* **38**, September 1999)

Notes
*   product known to damage latex

- **Progestogens** are compounds with progestogenic activity. They are added to oestrogen therapy (oral, transdermal and by implant) to protect against the development of endometrial hyperplasia and carcinoma (*Tables 2.6–2.9*). They can be used on their own to relieve vasomotor symptoms (*Table 2.18*).
- **Progestogen-only HRT** is an option for women with vasomotor symptoms in whom oestrogens are unwanted or contraindicated (see *Table 2.18*).
- **Progesterone** is the natural ovarian progestogen. It is poorly absorbed by mouth but is active if given by injection or in suppositories and pessaries. There are no routine uses for progesterone in the change. Its principal use is as an adjunct to fertility treatment.

- **Progest cream** is a yam derived form of progesterone in cream form marketed as a transdermal systemic progesterone alternative to oestrogen HRT. There is no peer reviewed data in the scientific literature on the product. It is promoted to women directly through periodicals and newspapers. A small prospective randomised double-blind placebo controlled crossover trial using higher doses of Progest than the product literature advises, found that it was possible to measure a rise in serum progesterone. However, the rise was so slight that any meaningful effect was unlikely. In addition to the exaggerated claims that have been made for Progest Cream, the product literature contains unsubstantiated and erroneous information about the detrimental effects of oestrogen HRT. 'Progest is unlikely to have any biological effects on bone and the endometrium at recommended doses' (Seeley, 1997; Cooper A, 1998).

- **Sequential progestogens** are a constituent of various HRT products. The progestogen is given for 10–14 days depending on formulation. They can be in combination with the oestrogen or come as a separate pill (*Tables 2.6–2.7*). Three progestogens are licensed for use with oestrogens which would otherwise be unopposed (Micronor HRT, Duphaston HRT and Crinone gel, see *Table 2.9*).

- **Transdermal progestogen:** Transdermal progestogens are currently available as norethisterone (Evorel Sequi, Evorel Conti, Estracombi) and levonorgestrel (Nuvelle TS).

Key issues in the use of progestogens as HRT:

- **adverse symptoms may be physical** (eg. cramps, acne, mastalgia, greasiness, flushes, weight gain) or psychological (eg. depression, irritability, panic attacks, anxiety, aggression). Many mimic premenstrual symptoms. Therapeutic options include reducing the dose or duration of the progestogen, changing to a formulation with a different progestogen or choosing an alternate route for delivery. Formulation, dose and duration data are listed in *Tables 2.6–2.9 and 2.13*.

- **breast disorder** has been alluded to as an adverse physical symptom of progestogen therapy. There has also been much interest in the role, if any, of progestogens in breast cancer among HRT users. The current consensus is that progestogens do not influence the risk of breast cancer in oestrogen HRT users. Data on breast disease incidence in continuous combined HRT users is awaited with interest.

- **lipid profiles** in oestrogen HRT users are adversely affected by the addition of a progestogen to the regime. Total cholesterol and LDL rise, HDL drops but so too do triglycerides. Recent data from the nurses' health study has however found that the addition of a progestogen does not have a detrimental effect on coronary artery disease risk (Grodstein *et al*, 1996). See *Table 2.4*.

Tibolone

Box 2.3: Tibolone therapy data

Indications: Period-free relief of vasomotor symptoms in non-hysterectomised women. It may also be useful in depressed mood, decreased libido and osteoporosis prevention

Cautions: Diabetes mellitus (diminishes glucose tolerance), lipid anomalies, renal dysfunction, epilepsy and migraine

Contraindications: Premenopausal use, cardio/cerebrovascular disease, hormone dependent tumour, severe liver disease, undiagnosed vaginal bleeding, pregnancy

Interactions: Enzyme inducing drugs (eg. phenytoin, carbamazepine, rifampicin) accelerate metabolism of tibolone, decreasing its effect. Tibolone enhances fibrinolytic activity which may affect anticoagulant activity

Tibolone (Livial) is a gonadomimetic compound combining oestrogenic, progestogenic and weak androgenic activity and is licensed for relief of menopausal symptoms and the prevention of osteoporosis. It is taken every day with no breaks in treatment. As with oestrogen continuous combined HRT, it should only be given to women who are twelve months past their menopause. It does not need to be balanced with a progestogen. Tibolone has no contraceptive effects. Changing from oestrogen containing HRT to tibolone should be preceded by a week or two of a progestogen. Oestrogen HRT can promote development of the endometrium which should be shed by using the progestogen before commencing tibolone. See *Table 2.8*.

SERMs

Box 2.4: SERM therapy data

Indications: Prevention of non-traumatic vertebral fractures in postmenopausal women at increased risk of osteoporosis

Cautions: Ensure calcium intake is adequate

Contraindications: History of venous thromboembolic events, prolonged immobilisation, hepatic or severe renal impairment, undiagnosed vaginal bleeding, endometrial or breast cancer

Interactions: Systemic oestrogens, cholestyramine

Selective estrogen/oestrogen receptor modulators have been around in the form of tamoxifen for some time. Tamoxifen has an oestrogen antagonistic effect on the breast but has agonist effects on the endometrium. Recently it was found that it also had agonist effects on bone and then the hunt was on for a more selective receptor modulator, ie. one that was antagonistic to endometrium as well as breast. The first of the second generation SERMs became available in Autumn 1998 in the UK. Raloxifene (Evista) is indicated for use in women at risk of vertebral fracture and will, over time, increase bone mineral density. It does not stimulate the endometrium so progestogen opposition is not required.

Unlike oestrogen, HRT appears to have a protective effect on breast tissue reducing the background risk of breast cancer, perhaps by as much as 50% (data from 21st Annual San Antonio Breast Cancer Symposium, 1998). Raloxifene is a viable alternative to bisphosphinates and especially oestrogens in women with osteoporosis who may be disinclined to taking oestrogens in their sixties or seventies. Raloxifene can cause menopausal type flushing and like oestrogen is associated with venous thromboembolism (see 'Oestrogen and SERMs; a comparison' *Table 2.11*.)

Table 2.11: SERMs and oestrogens; a comparison

Site of action	Oestrogen	SERM
Bone mineral density	increases BMD	increases BMD
Breast	small increased risk of cancer	probable substantially reduced cancer risk
Uterus	stimulates proliferation and risk of hyperplasia, atypia and carcinoma. Smaller increase in risk ifprogesten opposition	no stimulatory effect on endometrium
Vasomotor symptoms	abolished	hot flushes and sweats can be a minor effect
Venous thromboembolism	occasional	occasional
CVS	indirect studies suggest potential benefit (lipids, HDL2-C etc)	no data but overall beneficial effect on cholesterol, fibrinogen, triglycerides etc
CNS	may have protective effect against Alzheimer's disease	no data

(Ref: Walsh *et al*, 1998)

Table 2.12: HRT: Hormonal implants

Hormone	Dose	Delivery	Osteoporosis licence	Notes
Oestradiol (Organon)	25 mg 50 mg 100 mg	by implantation under local anaesthesia using trochar	Yes	i Check oestrogen levels before each implantation ii Tachyphylaxis known to occur iii Oestrogen effect on endometrium persists for a considerable length of time after last implant
Testosterone (Organon)	100 mg	by implanation under local anaesthesia using trochar	No data	i Used as adjunct to oestrogen implant HRT ii Usual dose 50–100 mg every 4–8 months iii Principal use in improving libido

Note: Trochar insertion kits may be purchased from Organon
Effect on latex is important to women using latex based contraceptive methods, eg. condoms and diaphragms.
Significant absorption of oestrogens by male partners of vaginal oestrogen users have been reported.
Oestrogen creams can be absorbed through the penile skin during vaginal intercourse and cases of gynaecomastia are on record.

Table 2.13: Progestogen choices

Progesten	2nd generation	3rd generation
Progesterone derived	dydrogesterone medroxyprogesterone	
Testosterone derived	norgestrel levonorgestrel norethisterone	desogestrel gestodene norgestimate

Notes: The **third generation progestogens** are all derivatives of norgtestrel and are said to be more progestagenic and less androgenic; however...
Only **second generation progestogens** are available in licensed HRT formulations
The **choice of progesten** depends on whether a more or less androgenic progesten is required. Acne, greasy hair and skin more common with androgenic derived progestens
Side effects of progestogens tend to be idiosyncratic. Swapping to another progestogen in the same class may help, eg. with breast tenderness. Alternatively, swapping to another class, eg. from testosterone to a progesterone derived compound may be effective

Table 2.14: Non-hormonal topical vaginal preparations

Astroglide	available by post. Data awaited
KY jelly	a traditional lubricant
Replens	non-hormonal aqueous vaginal moisturiser. One applicator full thrice weekly
Senselle	like Replens, Senselle is available over the counter at pharmacies

Calcium

Box 2.5: Calcium therapy data

Indications: Calcium deficiency; established osteoporosis in arresting or slowing down bone demineralisation

Cautions: Mild hypercalciuria, mild renal failure, treatment with thiazide diuretics

Contraindications: Hypercalcaemia, eg. in hyperparathyroidism, hypercalciuria, renal calculi, serum calcium raising tumours, eg. plasmocytoma and secondary bone tumours, severe renal failure, vitamin D overdosage

Interactions: Tetracyclines, fluorides, thiazide diuretics, theoretical interaction with digoxin

Unlike the hormonal methods used around the menopause which have vasomotor, psychological, urogenital, cardiovascular and skeletal benefits calcium and the biphosphinates only have a role in the prevention and treatment of osteoporosis. Calcium appears to be a very poor protector of skeletal mass in middle aged women. In the older woman who already has a degree of osteopaenia, calcium appears to slow down the rate of bone loss and may even promote a small increase in bone mass. Calcium supplements are essential in women taking biphosphinates and are advisable in women on long term steroid therapy. *Tables 2.15* and *2.16* list calcium preparations and the calcium content of various foodstuffs. One leading authority has suggested that post-menopausal women should have their own pint of milk each day; the calcium content of skimmed and semi-skimmed milk is the same as that in full cream milks. The advised daily intake of calcium is 800 mg increasing to 1 g in women over sixty years of age. If this cannot come from the diet, calcium supplements are advisable.

Table 2.15: Calcium preparations

Calcium salt	Product	Dose	Calcium content per dose	Pack size
gluconate	Non-Proprietary Non-Proprietary	tab eff 600 mg tab eff 1 g	53.4 mg 89 mg	20 100
carbonate	Calcit Calcichew Calcichew Forte Calcidrink Calcium-500	tab eff 1.25 g tab 1.25 g tab 2.5 g granules 2.52 g/sachet tab 1.25 g	500 mg 500 mg 1 g 1 g 500 mg	76 100 100 30 100
lactate	Non-Proprietary	tab 300 mg	39 mg	20
glubionate/ lactobionate	Calcium-Sandoz	syrup 5 ml= 1.09g/723 mg	108.3 mg/5 ml	500 ml
lactate gluconate/ carbonate	Sandocal-400	tab eff 930/700 mg	400 mg	5 x 20
lactate gluconate/ carbonate	Sandocal-1000	tab eff 2.327/1.75 g	1 g	3 x 10
hydroxyapatite	Ossopan 800 Ossopan granules	tab 830 mg granules 3.32 g/satchet	178 mg 712 mg	50 28
phosphate	Ostram	powder 3.3 g satchet	1.2 g	30

Principal sources: *MIMS*, November 1999; *BNF* **38**, September 1999

Notes:
Calcium will not prevent osteoporosis, however calcium supplements can be of benefit to women who have a marginal dietary intake **and** who have osteoporosis. In such cases, further bone loss may be slowed down or halted. It will not replace bone
Caution should be employed in prescribing calcium in the presence of renal impairment, sarcoidosis and thiazide diuretics. Calcium salts reduce the absorption of tetracyclines. See *Table 2.12* for dietary sources
Advised daily intake (dietary plus supplements) is 800mg rising to 1g for women over 60 years of age

Table 2.16: Calcium content of various foodstuffs

Product	Variety	Calcium content per 100g (mg)	Notes
Milk	pasteurised	115–20	1 pint = 450 g
	condensed/evaporated	330/290	
	soya	13	
Cheese	fromage frais	89	
	Blue Stilton	320	
	Cheddar/cheese spread	800/420	
	Brie	540	
	Edam	770	
Yoghurt	non-proprietary	140–200	small pot = 150 g
Choc ice	non-proprietary	130	
Rice pudding	canned	93	standard can circa 410 g
Cod	poached/fried	11/67	fried in sunflower oil
Haddock	steamed/fried	26/180	fried in sunflower oil
Mackerel	smoked/tinned in tomato sauce	20/82	
Salmon	steamed/smoked	23/19	
Sardines	canned in brine	540	
Whitebait	cooked in flour	860	
Prawns	boiled	110	
Fish...	cakes/fingers	150/92	
Bread	white/brown	120/110	
Crumpet	toasted	120	
Spaghetti	boiled	7	
Lasagne	boiled	6	
Rice	white/brown	18/4	boiled
Potatoes	boiled/instant with milk	5–24/44	
Baked beans	tinned in tomato sauce	48–55	
Lentils	boiled	22	
Mushy peas	tinned	14	
Spinach	boiled	160	high oxalate content
Cabbage	boiled	33	
Bacon	fried	7–16	depending on cut
Beef	cooked	6–15	depending on cut
Lamb	roast or grilled	7–9	more if bone scrapings present
Sausages	cooked	48–73	beef slightly higher calcium
Beef-burgers	fried	33	
Poultry	roast	9–12	grouse and partridge higher
Tripe	dressed/stewed	75/150	
Haggis	boiled	29	but first catch your Haggis

Notes:

Some experts advise post-menopausal women to have their own pint of milk delivered each day. The calcium content of skimmed and semi-skimmed is slightly higher than whole milk. Daily intake should probably be around 800 mg/day. Women over 60 are advised to have 1000 mg of calcium per day in their diet or as supplements. Studies quote 450–1500 mg/day. Most calcium should be present in the diet. In hard water areas, calcium will be absorbed in drinking water

Certain components of the diet can reduce the amount of calcium absorbed, eg. oxalates. So spinach which has a high calcium content is a poor source as it is mostly unavailable for absorption. Oxalates are also present in cocoa, chocolate and rhubarb, parsley, gooseberries, leeks, peanuts and peanut butter

Phytates also reduce the calcium absorbed

Diets that are very high in fats or fibre reduce the calcium available for absorption proteins

Neither oxalates nor phytates are problems if the overall diet is varied and mixed

Bisphosphinates

Box 2.6: Bisphosphinate therapy data

Indications: Reversal of established osteoporosis

Cautions: Renal impairment, renal calculi, where there is a risk of seizures, active upper GI problems, enterocolitis, Paget's disease of the bone

Contraindications: Severe renal impairment, hypercalcaemia, hypercalciuria, osteomalacia

Interactions: Food in the stomach reduces absorption as do calcium and other mineral preparations, possible increased GI events with NSAIDs and aspirin, the calcium phase of Didronel PMO may interfere with the absorption of tetracyclines. Severe hypocalcaemia has been reported with concurrent use of aminoglycoside antibiotics

These drugs promote the remineralisation of osteoporotic bone. They bind to calcium hydroxyappetite and inhibit bone reabsorption by osteoclasts. They are poorly absorbed and should be taken with water at least two hours before or after food. Biphosphinates can worsen osteomalacia. See *Table 2.17*.

Table 2.17: Biphosphinates

Drug/Indication	Product	Pack size	Administration	Inter-actions
alendronate sodium tablets (equivalent to 10 mg alendronic acid) indication: osteoporosis in postmenopausal women	Fosamax	30 days	I tab each morning with full glass of tap water 30 mins before food, drink or other medication. Contraindicated if GFR <35 ml/min	Calcium Antacids NSAIDs
disodium **etidronate** tablets 400 mg x 14 calcium carbonat tabs eff 1.25g x 76 indication: established vertebral osteoporosis	Didronel PMO	90 days	I etidronate tab/day x 2 weeks followed by I calcium tab/day x 76 consecutive days. Take etidronate tab in middle of 4-hour fast. Contraindicated in presence of hypercalcaemia, hypercalciuria, moderate or severe renal impairment and Paget's disease of the bone	

Notes:
Bisphosphonates are for the treatment of established osteoporosis not for its prevention
The BNF lists interactions with antacids, aminoglycoside antibiotics, iron and calcium salts

Biphosphinates are used in the treatment (not prevention) of established osteoporosis. Etidronate in the form of Didronel PMO is a cyclical therapy with a two week biphosphinate phase followed by 76 days of calcium supplementation. It is promoted as a treatment for established vertebral osteoporosis. Alendronate (Fosamax) is not cyclical, instead it is taken each day. It is promoted for treatment of osteoporosis at all sites. If required, calcium supplements can be taken at a different time of day to avoid interference with the absorption of the biphosphinate. Ideally, however, the manufacturers suggest correcting calcium and vitamin D deficiencies before treatment. The manufacturers of alendronate strongly advise users to wash the preparation down with a good volume of liquid; oesophageal ulceration has been reported. A third biphosphinate, sodium clodronate (Bonefos) is not licensed for use in osteoporosis.

Vaginal lubricants and non-hormonal options

See *Table 2.14* and *2.18*.

Contraception in the peri-menopause

Fertility at forty five years is 10 20/100 Women Years. This drops to around 5/HWY by fifty years. A serum FSH level 30 iu/l is generally accepted as the threshold above which in amenorrhoeic women over forty five years 'suggests' the menopause has been passed. The diagnosis of the menopause is retrospective and so contraception needs to be continued for twelve months after the last period. In this situation 'simple measures' are all that are required (barriers, spermicides). The situation is complicated if hormonal contraceptive methods are used.

- **Simple measures** are recommended in women with a history of amenorrhoea for less than one year and FSH30. They include barrier methods and spermicides (See *Tables 3.7* and *3.8*). Natural methods of family planning are not suitable because they rely on changes seen in cycling women.

- **The progestogen-only pill** does not suppress FSH or oestrogen depletion symptoms. Lengthening cycles or amenorrhoea are signs that ovarian activity may be waning. Two FSH levels 30u, at least one month apart, allow cessation of the POP and use of simple measures until 12 months since the final menstrual period. See *Table 3.4*.

- **The IUD:** Although copper IUDs begin to loose effectiveness after several years of use, fertility in the over forties declines more quickly. This results in a lower failure rate in the older IUD user. Copper IUDs fitted after the age of forty can be left in utero until after the change. They should be removed six months after the last period as involution and cervical stenosis can make removal more troublesome later. See *Table 3.6*.

- **The combined oral contraceptive pill** may be used by healthy non-smoking women without contraindications (squeaky clean) and who do not have a thrombophylic tendency, until the mid/late forties. The COC pill will mask the menopause and suppress pituitary FSH levels which only reliably rise to their true unsuppressed levels three months after cessation of the pill. If menstruation continues after stopping the pill or FSH, adequate contraception needs to be continued with. If amenorrhoea supervenes and the FSH is 30 simple measures, eg. spermicides or barriers can be used. A 20 mcg pill is probably best in women over forty-five years of age. See *Tables 3.2* and *3.3*.

- **The levonorgestrel IUS** (Mirena). The LNG-IUS would appear to be an excellent choice for contraception in the peri-menopause. There are even suggestions that it would be a convenient way to provide progestogens in oestrogen HRT users (it is not licensed for this however). See *Chapter 3*.

- **Depot progestogens** like Depo-Provera have a skeletal demineralising potential and are therefore to be avoided after the age of forty-five.

- **HRT** itself is not contraceptive, nor does it enhance fertility.

Table 2.18: Other treatments used in the change

Drug	Notes
norethisterone	5 mg/day can relieve flushes and sweats
medroxyprogesterone acetate	50–100 mg im every 1–2 months has been reported as effective for vasomotor symptoms
megestrol acetate	(NB **not** mestranol) 20–80 mg/day used in hot flushes with good effect
clonidine	25–75 mcg twice daily has given relief from flushes. Large placebo effect suspected
propranolol	may be helpful in palpitation. Diagnostic ECG etc advisable
naloxone	limited data
ethamsylate	250 mg QDS can reduce hot flushes
testosterone	poor response when compared with oestrogens/testosterone combined
nandrelone	androgen, used in osteoporosis. Not recommended in BNF
methyldopa	limited data
evening primrose oil	one comparative study found placebos were slightly better for vasomotor flushing
calcitriol	Vit D analogue used in osteoporosis. Careful investigation and monitoring. Caution in renal impairment
homeopathy	Numerous agents from aurum metallicum to valeriana can be prescribed depending on the particular mix of symptoms. An expert should be consulted
complementary therapies acupuncture, aromatherapy, Shiatsu	Apparently everything works for menopausal symptoms (according to complementary therapists)

Notes:
If any of the above therapies are considered, the BNF should be consulted first. Many of the treatments have been shown to have beneficial effects. However, their product licences may not cover use in the change

Useful Addresses:

- Amarant Trust
  80 Lambeth Road
  London SE1 7PW
- British Menopause Society
  83 High Street
  Marlow SL7 1AB
- National Osteoporosis Society
  PO Box 10, Radstock, Bath BA3 3YB

Recommended reading

Whitehead M, Godfree V (1992) *Hormone replacement therapy: your questions answered*. Churchill Livingstone, Edinburgh

References

Colditz GA *et al* (1995) The use of estrogens and progestens and the risk of breast cancer in postmenopausal women. *New Engl J Med* **332**:1589–93

The Collaborative Group on Hormone Factors in Breast Cancer (1997) Breast cancer and hormone replacement therapy: collaborative reanalysis of data from 51 epidemiological studies of 52,705 women with breast cancer and 108,411 women without breast cancer. *Lancet* **350**:1042–1043

Cooper A *et al* (1998) Systemic absorption of progesterone from Progest cream in postmenopausal women. *Lancet* **351**:1255–6

Davidson N (1995) Hormone-replacement therapy – breast versus heart versus bone. *New Engl J Med* **332**:1638–9

Drugs and Therapeutics Bulletin (1999) Drugs in the peri-operative period: 3 — Hormonal contraceptives and hormone replacement therapy. *Drug Ther Bull* **37**: 78–80

Grady D *et al* (1992) Hormone therapy to prevent disease and prolong life in postmenopausal women. *Ann Intern Med* **117**:1016–37

Grodstein F *et al* (1996) Postmenopausal estrogen use and the risk of cardiovascular disease. *New Engl J Med* **335**:453–61

Hanggi W *et al* (1997) Long term influence of different postmenopausal hormone replacement regimes on serum lipids and lipoprotein (a): a randomised study. *Br J Obstet Gynaecol* **10**:708–717

Hulley S *et al* (1998) Randomized trial of estrogen plus progestin for secondary prevention of coronary heart disease in postmenopausal women. *JAMA* **280**: 605–613

Pereira Gray D *et al* (1995) HRT prescribing — a paradigm for the complexity of prescribing in general practice? *RCGP Year Book* 1995: 245–250

Postuma WFM *et al* (1994) Cardioprotective effects of hormone replacement therapy in postmenopausal women: is the evidence biased? *Br Med J* **308**: 268–9

Royal College of Obstetricians and Gynaecology (1999) *Hormone replacement therapy and venous thromboembolism*. RCOG Guideline, No 19: April

Seeley T (1997) Commenting on 'The absorption of progesterone from Progest cream' a presentation by Dr A Cooper, The Menopause Clinic, King's College Hospital, London. *J Brit Menopause Society* **3**:23

Stampfer MJ *et al* (1991) Postmenopausal estrogen therapy and cardiovascular disease. *New Engl J Med* **325**: 756–62

Tang M-X *et al* (1996) Effect of oestrogen during menopause on risk and age at onset of Alzheimer's disease. *Lancet* **348**: 429–32

Utian WH (1996) Direction, misdirection and misconception in menopause research and management. *Br J Obstet Gynaecol* **103**: 736–39

Walsh BW *et al* (1998) Effects of Raloxifene on serum lipids and coagulation factors in healthy postmenopausal women. *JAMA* **279**: 1445–1451

3
contraception

Contraceptive options are presented in this chapter. Detailed answers to commonly posed questions are listed alphabetically. Data can be located for each method by using the chapter contents and in the numerous tables and information boxes.

Chapter contents

Boxes

Tables

Combined oral contraceptive pill

See *Box 3.1*. Introduced over thirty years ago, the combined oral contraceptive pill is the commonest form of contraception used in the United Kingdom today. Around one fifth of women in this country use it in their fertile years and the figure rises to just under 50% for women in their early twenties.

Combined pill formulations are listed in *Tables 3.1* and *3.2*.

Box 3.1: The combined oral contraceptive pill

Indications: Reversible contraception (menstrual cycle control, primary dysmenorrhoea, post coital contraception, polycystic ovary syndrome)

Cautions: Cigarette smoking (avoid in women over 35 years), hypertension, obesity, diabetes mellitus (avoid if retinopathy or nephropathy present), family history of ischaemic heart disease or cerebrovascular accident (especially in relatives <45 years), varicose veins, severe depression, long term immobilisation, sickle cell disease, inflammatory bowel disease

Contraindications: Pregnancy, trophoblastic disease, major risk factors for arterial or venous thrombosis, valvular heart disease, pulmonary hypertension, severe hypertension, varicose veins under treatment or where thrombosis has occurred, lipid anomalies, known coagulopathy, focal crescendo or severe migraine, transient cerebral ischaemic attacks, liver disease, gall bladder disease, haemolytic uraemic syndrome, pregnancy occurrence of cholestasis, pemphigoid (herpes gestationalis) or deterioration in otosclerosis, breast or genital tract carcinoma, undiagnosed vaginal bleeding, unruptured cerebral aneurism or strong family history of cerebral arterial aneurism (*breast feeding, **altitude)

Interactions: Antihypertensive including ace inhibitors and beta-blockers (oestrogens antagonise hypotensive effect), antibacterials (i) broad spectrum **antibiotics** reduce contraceptive effect (ii) rifampicin accelerates metabolism of oestrogens and progestins, anticoagulant effects antagonised, antidepressants antagonised and tricyclic plasma levels increased, antidiabetic hypoglycaemic effects antagonised, **antiepileptics** (carbamazepine, phenobarbitone, phenytoin, primidone) accelerate oestrogen metabolism, **oral antifungals** griseofulvin and oral imidazoles? (fluconazole, itraconazole, ketoconazole), cyclosporin concentration increased, diuretic effects antagonsied, theophylline plasma concentrations increased by delayed excretion, spironolactone (enzyme induction)

Notes:

*Breast feeding listed as a contraindication to COC pill in BNF 'until weaning or for 6 months after birth'. See 'Key issues'

**The combined pill is also contraindicated in women travelling to (but not resident in and thoroughly acclimatised to) high altitudes because of increased blood viscosity and enhanced thrombotic tendency

- The above data also apply to 'phasic'combined pills
- If two or more 'cautions' are present, the COC pill should not be used
- Interactions in bold may lead to contraceptive failure

Table 3.1: Monophasic combined oral contraceptive pills

Oestrogen dose (mcg)	Progestin type	progestin dose (mg)	Product	Notes
20	NET	1.0	Loestrin 20	
20	DES *	0.15	Mercilon	
20	GEST	0.075	Femodette	
30	NET	1.5	Loestrin 30	
30	LNG	0.15	Microgynon 30	also as ED
30	LNG	0.15	Ovranette	
30	LNG	0.25	Eugynon 30	
30	LNG	0.25	Ovran 30	
30	DES *	0.15	Marvelon	
30	GEST *	0.075	Femodene	Also as ED
30	GEST *	0.075	Minulet	
35	CYPR	2.0	Dianette	acne/hirsutism
35	NET	0.5	Brevinor	
35	NET	0.5	Ovysmen	
35	NET	1.0	Neocon 1/35	
35	NET	1.0	Norimin	
35	NRGT	0.25	Cilest	
50	LNG	0.25	Ovran	
50	NET	1.0	Norinyl-1	E-mestranol

Principal sources: *MIMS*, November 1999; *BNF* **38**, September 1999

Notes:
* 3° generation progestogen containing pills
LNG levonorgestrel
NET norethisterone (and ethinodiol diacetate)
NRGT norgestimate (3° generation progestagen but behaves like a 2° generation after absorption and metabolism)
DES desogestrel
GEST gestodene
CYPR cyproterone acetate; a pregnane type anti-androgen (see 'Acne', *Chapter 1*)
ED 'everyday' packs include 7 dummy pills for week of withdrawal bleed

Pros and cons

See *Box 3.2*. Most women taking the combined pill do not experience detrimental side-effects. In fact, most gain benefits in addition to contraception.

Initial choice of product will depend on prescriber preference but *Boxes 3.3* and *3.4* may assist in choosing an appropriate pill for individuals with pre-existing tendencies and conditions. The information is helpful in the rational choice of an alternative when one product has produced hormonal side-effects.

Table 3.2: Bi/triphasic combined oral contraceptive pills

Phase	Ethinyl-oestradiol dose (mcg)	Progestin	Dose (mg)	Product	Notes
Biphasic	35/35	NET	0.5–1	Binovum	
Triphasic Triphasic	35/35/35 35/35/35	NET NET	0.5–1–0.5 0.5–0.75–1	Synphase TriNovum	
Triphasic Triphasic	30/40/30 30/40/30	LNG LNG	0.05–0.075–0.125 0.05–0.075–0.125	Logynon Trinordiol	also as ED
Triphasic Triphasic	30/40/30 30/40/30	GEST * GEST *	0.05–0.07–0.1 0.05–0.07–0.1	Triadene Triminulet	

Principal sources: *MIMS*, November 1999; *BNF* **38**, September 1999

Notes:

Oestrogen ethinyloestradiol except Orth Novin 1/50 which contains mestranol

*	3° generation progestogen containing pills
LNG	Levonorgestrel
NET	norethisterone (and ethinodiol diacetate)
DES	desogestrel
GEST	gestodene
ED	'everday' packs include 7 dummy pills for week of withdrawal bleed

Box 3.2: Pros and cons of the combined oral contraceptive pill

Benefits of the combined pill	Major side-effects of the combined pill
contraception cycle stabilisation/control *less...* menorrhagia dysmenorrhoea premenstrual symptoms acne and hirsutism *reduced risk of...* ovarian cysts ovarian cancer endometriosis endometrial cancer uterine fibroids benign breast disease iron deficiency salpingitis rheumatoid arthritis(?)	venous thromboembolism arterial thrombosis (coronary, cerebral mesenteric etc) subarachnoid haemorrhage hypertension cholelithiasis depression *increased neoplasia* breast cancer liver, benign and malignant

Box 3.3: Potential hormonal side-effects of the combined oral contraceptive pill

Oestrogen side-effects	Progestogen side-effects
breast enlargement and tenderness bloating weight gain (fluid retention) carpal tunnel syndrome headaches vaginal moistness nausea, chloasma	acne hirsuitism weight gain (increased appetite) depression decreased libido vaginal dryness greasy hair

Box 3.4: Hormonal dominance of various combined oral contraceptive pills

Oestrogen dominant pills	Progestogen dominant pills	Neutral
Brevinor Ovysmen Neocon 1/35 Norimin Trinovum ** Ovran ** Norinyl-1 ** Ortho Novin 1/50	Loestrin 20 Loestrin 30 Microgynon/Ovranette Trinordiol/Logynon	Cilest * Triadene/* Triminulet * Marvelon * Minulet/* Femodene * Mercilon

Notes:
Full details of all combined pills are found in *Tables 3.1* and *3.2*
* signifies third generation pill
** signifies 50 mcg oestrogen pills
Neutral pills are listed in decreasing oestrogen dominance
For women with oestrogen side-effects, choose a lower dose oestrogen pill or swap to a more progestin dominant pill and vice versa
Dianette (ethinyloestradiol/cyproterone acetate) not included

Key issues and the combined oral contraceptive pill

Women taking contraceptive precautions generally do so when in good health. The occurrence of side-effects is therefore less tolerable than in those taking drugs for illness. The principle of relative risk applies in both situations, though in the case of illness it is easier to appreciate. The significance of relative risk has been highlighted by the recent controversy over the third generation progestogen containing pills. The risks of a particular pill should not be compared with nothing, but with the alternatives. See *Box 3.5* for major risk factors.

Every woman (or couple) presenting for contraceptive assistance is individual and requires particular advice. Indeed the same woman may have very different contraceptive requirements at different stages in her own life.

● **Age and the pill**: fecundity, the ability to conceive in any one cycle, decreases with age. This has the effect of making all forms of contraception more reliable as a woman gets older. In women with no apparent risk factors the combined pill can be used until the menopause. Thromboembolic disorder and breast cancer are age linked, making use of the pill from the mid-forties onwards contentious. The lowest effective dose of oestrogen and progestogen should be chosen.

The oestrogen component of the pill will mask the menopause. The only way to diagnose the passing of the menopause is to stop the pill and observe while using alternative contraceptive precautions. Serum FSH estimations can aid diagnosis, but only if the pill is stopped for a few weeks. A level >30iu/l is suggestive of the climacteric, especially if a repeat some time later is also raised. If menstruation resumes after stopping the pill, then ovulation and fertility are distinct possibilities.

Contraceptive precautions are advised for two years after the menopause, but simple measures may well be satisfactory. An IUD or the levonorgestrel IUS are valuable alternatives.

- **Amenorrhoea after the pill**: the combined pill is blamed for many things, not least post-pill amenorrhoea and infertility. The truth, however, is that women with menstrual or fertility problems after the pill either had them before taking the pill or were predisposed to and destined to get one of these common conditions anyway. (One study has shown reduced fecundity in older, nulliparous women who came off the combined pill. Ultimate fertility was unaffected)

- **Antibiotics and the pill**: certain broad spectrum antibiotics interfere with the contraceptive action of the pill by disturbing bowel flora. Bacteria are involved in the enterohepatic circulation of oestrogens. The consequence is that in some women plasma oestrogen levels drop and ovarian activity can resume. The most likely antibiotics with which this may happen are ampicillin and its derivatives, tetracyclines and the cephalosporins. It is not a problem with penicillin V or co-trimoxazole. There is some dispute about erythromycins: they appear to be unpredictable in their interference with the efficacy of the combined pill. Rifampicin has a potent and prolonged effect on pill reliability (see data sheet).

  Long term low dose antibiotic treatments, as may be used in the management of recurrent UTI or acne vulgaris, are however probably safe as the bowel flora re-establishes and the enterohepatic circulation normalises after a couple of weeks on treatment

- **Antifungals and the pill**: griseofulvin reduces the contraceptive effect of the combined pill. The oral imidazoles (fluconazole, itraconazole and ketoconazole) are listed in the *BNF* as 'causing pill failure in anecdotal reports'. The *ABPI Data Sheet Compendium* states that itraconazole does not interfere with the metabolism of ethinyloestradiol, that kinetic studies of multiple 50 mg doses of fluconazole did not have any relevant effect on hormone levels (although the 200 mg dose did) and that oral ketoconazole has been reported to have caused menstrual irregularity in women using the combined pill. The topical imidazoles (clotrimazole, miconazole etc) are not listed as posing a risk to the pill but some can damage latex

Box 3.5: Risk factors and the combined oral contraceptive pill

Women at increased risk of major side-effects on combined pill
smokers
older women
obese women
diabetes mellitus
hypertensive women
familial hyperlipidaemia
family history of breast cancer
personal or family history of thromboembolic disorder

- **Breakthrough bleeding** may be caused by using a pill with too low a dose of oestrogen or progestogen. It is mandatory to exclude abnormal vaginal bleeding before experimenting with alternative pill formulations. 'Apparent' breakthrough bleeding can be caused by genital tract cancer, especially from the cervix, as well as by disturbances in pregnancy. Gastrointestinal upset may reduce absorption enough to cause erratic bleeding. Vegetarians are said to be more prone to it because the intestinal flora involved in the enterohepatic circulation of oestrogens may be deficient. More importantly, drug interactions must be considered.

  Missed pills are a common cause of breakthrough bleeding. However, mild breakthrough bleeding in the absence of poor compliance probably does not imply poor contraceptive cover. If breakthrough bleeding is persistent, changing to a phased formulation can be tried. A pill with a higher or different dose of progestogen can be tried, as can a 50 mcg oestrogen pill. But always beware of missing serious pathology

- **Breast disease** is common with a lifetime risk for its development being around 1:12. It is commoner in women with a strong family history (first degree relative who developed cancer before the age of fifty) and the combined pill is strongly contraindicated in such women. Breast cancer is more common in women with benign breast disease and this too is a relative contraindication. The protective effect of the COC pill against the development of benign breast disease is a separate issue.

  A recent retrospective Dutch study suggests that the incidence of breast cancer, although not raised overall compared with non-users, was higher in women who began the pill in their teens and older current users (46–54 years). 'Ever use' before the age of 20 carried a relative risk of developing cancer before the age of 36 years of 3.5 (p>0.01) (Rookus and van Leeuwen, 1994). The UK National Case Control Study (1989) stated that the background risk of a woman developing breast cancer before the age of 36 was 2:1000. In COC pill users it was 3:1000. Against this the benefits of the pill must be balanced

- **Cervical dysplasia and cancer**: no direct link to cervical dysplasia and malignancy has been shown. Cervical cancer is more common among women who commence sexual intercourse at an early age, who have numerous sexual partners, who have been infected with the human papilloma virus and who use non-barrier methods of contraception. In other words, the link between the pill and cervical cancer appears casual not causal. Women with intraepithelial neoplasia can continue using the pill

- **Diabetes mellitus** is a strong relative contraindicationto the pill. In the presence of other risk factors it is contraindicated especially with microvascular disease, hypertension or smoking. Professor Guillebaud (1994) advises using the combined pill with great caution for short periods of time and only in young diabetics totally free of any complication or contraindication, and where there is no satisfactory alternative.

  Pointers of future risk of diabetes (eg. strong family history, gestational diabetes or a previous macrosomic infant) are not contraindications to the pill but care should be employed in monitoring patients, particularly with regard to weight. The lowest dose pill formulation should be chosen

- **Epilepsy** is not caused and is rarely exacerbated by the pill. Certain antiepileptic drugs are enzyme inducing agents and will reduce the effectiveness of the pill. These drugs are barbiturates, carbamazepine, phenytoin and primidone. The newer anti-convulsants lamotrigine, vigabantin as well as sodium valproate and the benzodiazepine clonazepam are exceptions and are safe to use with the pill (Szarewski and Guillebaud, 1994).

Seizure control is improved with a steady hormonal pattern. Monophasics are therefore recommended in women with epilepsy. It is also recommended that tri-cycle regimes be employed with a shortened pill-free interval. (See below, and do not confuse with triphasic formulations). In addition to smoother hormonal delivery it is also essential to give an adequate dose of oestrogen. In women on enzyme inducing anti-convulsants at least 50 mcg is required each day. If poor cycle control occurs, or if there is breakthrough bleeding, up to 100 mcg per day can be given by taking more than one pill per day, eg. a 30+30 mcg, 35+50 mcg, 50+50 mcg dose

- **Failure of contraception** associated with the COC pill is low (0.1–3.0/100 women years). Failure is increased in certain definite situations: **pill omission** (especially on either side of the pill free interval); **drug interaction** (eg. broad spectrum antibiotics, anticonvulsants, rifampicin), **gastrointestinal disorder** (acute gastro/enteritis, inflammatory bowel disease). Recently, new guidelines have been issued on action to be taken if pill(s) have been missed (see *Table 3.3*)

Table 3.3: Advice for women forgetting combined pill taking

For single pill omissions of less than 12 hours:	Take the missed pill straight away and further pills as usual
For one or more pill omissions and more than 12 hours late:	
... in 'week one' of the pill packet	Take the last pill straight away. Continue with the packet as usual. If SI has not occurred in the last 7 days use a barrier for next 7 days. If SI has occurred see a doctor as EC may be required
... in 'week two' of the pill packet	Take the last pill straight away. Continue with the packet as usual. If four or more pills have been missed, use a barrier as well for next 7 days
... in 'week three' of the pill packet	Take the last pill straight away. Continue with the packet as usual. At the end of the packet continue without a break with next packet. BTB may occur. An alternative would be to stop taking pills until seven pill free days have transpired and start the next packet then

(Ref: Korver T *et al*, 1995)

Notes:
EC   emergency contraception
SI   sexual intercourse
BTB   breakthrough bleeding

- **Fertility after stopping the pill** is considered to be unaffected. It is possible that in older nulliparous women fecundity (the ability to conceive per cycle) may be lower, but fertility (the ability to conceive) is not affected

- **Gall bladder disease** is probably slightly higher in pill users. Evidence from a nurses' health study in the United States found that obesity was most strongly associated with risk (Grodstein *et al*, 1994). The combined pill carried a relative increase in risk of 1.2 (95% CI 0.9–1.5)

- **Heart disease and the pill**: coronary artery disease, high risk of coronary artery disease, cardiomyopathy and pulmonary hypertension are all absolute contraindications to the COC pill. The incidence of myocardial infarction appears to be higher in second compared with third generation pill users. The statistical significance of benefit using third generation pills in the study by Lewis (1996) was weak

- **Hypertension** can be caused by the pill and, if pre-existing, is a relative contraindication to its use. Toxaemia in pregnancy is a special form of hypertensive disorder that appears to be especially significant as a risk factor mitigating against use of the combined pill. A past history of toxaemia and pill use significantly increases the risk of developing coronary artery disease

- **Inflammatory diseases** are relative contraindications. Both ulcerative colitis and Crohn's disease are inflammatory disorders and are therefore attended with a higher risk of venous thrombosis. Other inflammatory disorders, of which rheumatoid arthritis and systemic lupus erythematosis are perhaps the most important, are relatively contraindicated because of their enhanced thrombotic potential. Curiously, the combined pill may offer a degree of protection against the development of rheumatoid arthritis

- **Initiation of oral contraception**: current advice is to start on the first day of a period. This gives immediate contraception. Commence on the second day if there is doubt whether the bleed is a period. Traditionally COC pills were commenced on Day 5 of the cycle. This gives good cycle control, but contraceptive cover is slow (precautions are needed for seven further days after starting).

  Transfer from one formulation to another depends on the dose of hormones in the two products. If the previous pill was of a higher or equivalent dose then a swap omitting the pill free interval gives continuity of contraception. If the previous pill was a lower dose, then the seven day break can be observed with continuity of contraception.

  Manufacturers of third generation pills advised additional contraceptive precautions for the first seven days on a second generation pill if a seven day break had occurred. They recommended two weeks of additional precautions in cases where a swap from a third generation ED (everyday) to a second generation ED formulation was made even when both the pill free week or dummy tablets were avoided (Schering, 1995). After miscarriage, the combined pill can be started immediately.

  In non-lactating women, commencement is not advised sooner than 21 days after delivery because of the enhanced thrombolic risks. See 'Lactation'

- **Lactation** is adversely affected by the combined pill. Milk quality and yield may be affected and some hormone will transfer via the milk to the baby. This constitutes a relative contraindication to the combined pill. The immediate postpartum phase constitutes a relative thromboembolic risk time which also militates against the COC pill. Postpartum starting regimes generally advise waiting until after the sixth week, although some have advocated starting after 2–3 weeks and others 12 weeks postpartum. Pills containing norethisterone are best avoided as a significant amount of the hormone transfers to the milk (unlike levonorgestrel)

- **Legal matters in under 16-year-olds**: in 1985 five Law Lords decided by a vote of three to two that under certain circumstances doctors may give contraceptive advice and prescriptions to girls under the legal age of consent, and rejected Mrs Victoria Gillick's appeal that parental consent could not be dispensed with. The guidelines are:
  - that the girl, although under 16 years of age, will understand (the doctor's) advice
  - that (the doctor) cannot persuade her to inform her parents or allow (the doctor) to inform the parents that she is seeking contraceptive advice
  - that she is very likely to begin or continue having sexual intercourse with or without contraceptive treatment
  - that unless she receives contraceptive advice or treatment her physical or mental health, or both, are likely to suffer
  - that her best interests require (the doctor) to give her contraceptive advice, treatment or both without the parental consent (Dyer, 1985).

Medical confidentiality rules apply to these as in other matters

- **Migraine** is a family of disorders. Focal migraine, crescendo migraine, severe migraine requiring ergot treatment and importantly, migraine that develops or deteriorates after the COC pill is commenced, are absolute contraindications to the pill. Professor Guillebaud also includes sumatriptan users in the absolute contraindication category as this drug is a vasoconstrictor which may add to the thrombotic risks of the pill (Guillebaud J, 1994). Migraine must be distinguished from common headache.

  Some women get so called 'menstrual migraine' and headaches. These may improve if the pill is given with fewer pill-free intervals (tri-cycling; see below)

- **Missed pill advice** is summarised in *Table 3.3*

- **Older women and the combined pill**: provided there are no contraindications whatsoever to the combined pill and that the woman prefers it to alternatives, then it is permissible to prescribe the pill up until the menopause. Hypertension, obesity and smoking are the commonest reasons not to prescribe the pill to older women (see section above; 'Age and the pill')

- **Otosclerosis** can be made worse by the pill (and by HRT). The combined pill should be prescribed with great caution if no other method is acceptable. It should not be prescribed if there has been a previous deterioration in pregnancy

- **Pill-free interval**. This is traditionally set at seven days. There is no compelling scientific or biological reason for this. There are moves to make available pill formulations with shorter pill-free intervals which will reduce the risk of contraceptive failure. It is generally reckoned that around ten pill-free days increase significantly the risk of ovulation. The seven regular pill-free days can be effectively extended by pill omission on either side of the break. Mid-cycle omissions are for that reason less risky than just before or after the week off.

  Some women get adverse symptoms in their pill-free week (eg. migraine, convulsions). In such women 'tri-cycle' regimes (see below) and four-day pill-free intervals have much to recommend them

- **Rifampicin** is a potent enzyme-inducer and even brief exposure can interfere with the contraceptive effect of the combined pill for a month. It is used in the treatment of tuberculosis but will be more commonly encountered as prophylaxis following meningococcus exposure. Prolonged alternative contraceptive measures are essential

- **Sickle cell disease** is a condition associated with thrombotic episodes and stroke. Pregnancy is a particularly hazardous time for affected women. The COC pill also poses its own thrombotic risk which makes the pill a strong relative contraindication in sickle cell disease. Depot progestogens are usually the preferred option. Heterozygous carriers of the sickle cell trait can use the pill

- **Smoking** is the largest preventable cause of coronary artery disease in the UK today. The pill also increases the risk of coronary artery disease. The two risks combined, especially in older women or women with hypertension, so increase the risks that the pill is contraindicated. Cigarette smoking in women under 35 years is a relative contraindication to using the COC pill

- **Splenectomy** of itself is not a contraindication to the COC pill. If, however, it was performed for a reason that would preclude COC pill use, or if in any circumstance the platelet count rises to unacceptable levels ($>500 \times 10^9$/L) then the COC pill should not be used

- **Surgery and the combined pill**: the risk here is venous thromboembolic disease. Pill users should stop taking their pill at least four weeks before major surgery or minor surgery if it involves the legs (eg. arthroscopy of the knee), the veins of the leg or if immobilisation will follow the operation. Minor procedures otherwise should not require cessation of the pill. In women requiring emergency surgery (eg. appendectomy or orthopaedic procedures) and who are on the pill, the pill should be stopped and heparin given. The pill is not recommenced until at least two weeks after full mobilisation (Guillebaud, 1994)

- **Teenage contraception**: although the COC pill is a highly effective method and may well be indicated in highly fertile young women it is not without its particular drawbacks. These relate to reliability of taking the pill regularly, and exposure to seminal fluid:
  - although precision in time of taking is not as critical as with the POP, it is still important
  - seminal fluid, in addition to carrying the risk of pregnancy can also carry sexually transmitted diseases. These are more likely in women who are not in monogamous stable relationships
  - the juvenile cervix which may not have completed squamous metaplasia is vulnerable to neoplastic influences. To protect against this and STD, young women COC pill users are advised to employ a barrier method (usually condoms) in addition to oral contraception

- **Teratogenesis** is not listed in association with the COC pill in the *BNF*. However, there have been reports of genital developmental anomalies. A large meta-analysis found the risk of external male genital developmental anomaly (hypospadias, cryptorchidism) to be marginally raised (Rauman-Wilms *et al*, 1995). The relative risk overall was 1:11 but with wide confidence intervals crossing unity (95% CI 0.04–29.21). The effect, if anything, is minimal. It is thought that the COC pill is taken in around 1:40 early pregnancies

- **Third generation pills** are ones containing the progestogens, gestodene or desogestrel. Norgestimate is a third generation progestogen but is metabolised to and behaves as a second generation progestogen. In Autumn 1995, the Committee on the Safety of Medicines advised doctors that there was a doubling of the tiny risk of venous thromboembolism in third generation pill users compared with second generation pill users. This advice was confirmed (Spitzer, 1996). The overall risk of non-fatal DVT/PE in women not using the pill is around 5–11/100,000 women per year. In pregnancy that risk rises to 60/100,000 per year. The risks attributed to second and third generation pills are 15 and 30/100,000 women per year respectively.

  The Scientific Committee of the Faculty of Family Planning and Reproductive Health Care (1996) recommend initiation of the third generation COC pill be restricted to women who have a medical indication such as acne or hirsutism (third generation pills appear less androgenic), where there is user preference for a third generation pill and where the woman is fully acquainted with the thrombo-embolic risks and is without other contraindications.

  Since October 1995 there has been increasing evidence that the higher thrombo-embolic risks of the third generation pills may be spurious. Prescribing habits before the 'pill scare' may have lead to preferential prescribing to women with risk factors and new pill users; both groups with a higher thrombo-embolic potential. In other words, selection bias may account for the figures. This is further reassurance for those women who wish to take or transfer back to third generation pills.

  Third generation pills may be attended by less arterial thrombotic risk in the form of myocardial infarction. What risks to the vasculature that do attend the use of the pill are as nothing compared with smoking cigarettes

- **Thromboembolic disorder** is an absolute contraindication to the use of the combined pill

- **Thrombophilia** or an increased tendency to thrombose is more common in the population than has previously been realised. It is often familial. In one American study the population incidence of the heterozygous form of the commonest thrombophilia, Factor V Leiden mutation, was 7%. Dutch and Swedish studies have found slightly lower incidences. If it is proposed to give the pill to someone with a family history of venous thromboembolism, a thrombophilia screen and exclusion of the Leiden mutation is recommended

- **Tri-cycling regimes** involve taking three 21-day monophasic pill packets back-to-back without a break. The advantages include, less frequent withdrawal bleeding and better contraceptive cover. The pill-free week is a time of heightened risk of failure; the fewer the breaks the lower the risk of pregnancy. Breakthrough bleeding is slightly commoner than with single cycle regimes, but many women prefer the overall convenience of the method.

  Women with epilepsy are advised to 'tri-cycle' as it keeps hormone levels more steady reducing hormone fluctutation induced convulsions. In addition, the pill-free interval can be shortened to five or even four days.

  Breakthrough bleeding is an occasional nuisance

- **Varicose veins and thrombophlebitis**: varicose veins are not a contraindication to the use of the pill in women who wish to use it. However, varicose veins can be a marker of other contraindicating conditions, eg. obesity or previous DVT. Thrombophlebitis is a contraindication to the pill as it signifies a thrombotic tendency unless a totally reassuring thrombophylia screen is found

---

Progestogen-only pill

See *Box 3.6*. The progesterone-only pills (POP) are the only oral contraceptives that are oestrogen free. They have several possible modes of action. Not only do women differ in the way the POP works for them, but the same woman may respond differently at various times to the same formulation. In some women the effect is principally on cervical mucus. These women will tend to maintain their usual cycle as the pituitary ovarian axis is unaffected. At the other extreme some women's ovaries are effectively switched off and they become amenorrhoeic. Contraception is principally provided here by anovulation. In between lie women with varying degrees of ovarian functional interference from mild effects on the luteal (progesterone) phase to interference with the follicular development phase. These women may have frequent and erratic vaginal bleeding. Interestingly, it is the women with regular cycles who are at most risk of POP contraceptive failure.

Progestogen-only pill formulations are listed in *Table 3.4*.

Box 3.6: The progestogen-only pill

Indications: Contraception

Cautions: Hypertension, thromboembolic disorder, hormone dependent cancer including current trophoblastic disease, liver disease and recurrent cholestatic jaundice, functional ovarian cysts, focal migraine, malabsorption syndromes

Contraindications: Pregnancy and suspected pregnancy, undiagnosed abnormal vaginal bleeding, severe arterial disease and ischaemic heart disease, liver adenoma, porphyria, previous ectopic pregnancy

Interactions: Enzyme inducing drugs (i) antiepileptics; carbamazepine, phenobarbitone, phenytoin, primidone (ii) antibiotics; rifampicin and griseofulvin accelerate POP metabolism (iii) spironolactone; cyclosporin levels increased

---

Table 3.4: Progestogen-only contraceptive pills

Progestin type	Dose (mcg)	Product	Pack size
norethisterone	350	Micronor	28 x 3
	350	Noriday	28 x 3
	500	Femulen *	28
levonorgestrel	30	Microval	35
	30	Norgeston	35
	(75)	Neogest **	35

Principal sources: *MIMS*, November 1999; *BNF* **38**, September 1999

Notes:

*   ethinodiol acetate (norethisterone type)

**   norgestrel with 50% levonorgestrel and 50% an inactive isomer; dextronorgestrel

POP: key issues

● **Age**: all methods of contraception become more effective in older women as their fecundity decreases. The POP is no exception. Added to this are lower age-related side effects compared with the COC pill. Because the POP method requires precise regularity in pill taking it is often more suited to older women who tend to be less chaotic with their contraceptive arrangements

● **Amenorrhoea** occurs in around 1:6 women and indicates (in the absence of other causes of amenorrhoea which must be considered, eg. prolacinoma, pregnancy, menopause) that the ovaries are inactive. Women with amenorrhoea caused by the POP can be reassured that their failure rates are the lowest with this method of contraception. Prolonged amenorrhoea, say five years, especially in women who smoke should prompt the prescriber to assess bone mineral density. If this is satisfactory and if serum oestradiol levels are above 100 pmol/l the POP can be continued until the mid forties

● **Antibiotic use**: with the exception of the enzyme inducing drugs, rifampicin and griseofulvin, there is no interference with contraceptive cover. Some authorities advise giving more than one POP tablet each day if enzyme inducing drugs are being used

● **Blood pressure** is not affected by the POP

● **Cancer**: the POP has not been linked to the development of any cancers. It is, however, contraindicated in the hormone dependent cancers of breast and uterus as well as the gestational trophoblastic diseases (hydatidiform mole, choriocarcinoma)

● **Commencement regime**: usually started on day 1–2 of the cycle. POPs can though be started at any time if pregnancy is excluded and extra precautions are continued for seven days.

　　Postpartum commencement is usually on the 21st day. It can be later (up to 28 days) in lactators. Later starts should follow exclusion of pregnancy and extra precautions for seven days

- **Coronary artery disease** does not appear to be related to use of the POP

- **Diabetes mellitus** is not a contraindication to use of the POP. No alteration in insulin requirements should be seen

- **Emergency contraception** Levonorgestrel has been used for emergency contraception for several years (the Ho and Kwan method). A WHO study comparing it with the Yuzpe method found it more effective and attended by fewer side effects. For details see the section on 'Emergency contraception' below

- **Failure rates** vary with age at 3.1/100 women years in women aged 25–29 years to 0.3 for women over 40 years. Failures are also commoner among women who menstruate regularly on the POP. POP induced amenorrhoea confers the most effective contraception as it signifies ovarian inactivity. Failure rates are higher than the COC pill as timing of pill taking is crucial (see below: 'Timing')

- **Ectopic pregnancy** is not increased among users of the POP. However, because their principal effect is in prevention of intrauterine pregnancy, when 'breakthrough' pregnancy does occur proportionately more will be ectopic than in women who were not using contraception; ie. few ectopic but even fewer intrauterine pregnancies. The risk of breakthrough pregnancies being ectopic is similar to that seen with the IUD

- **Lactation** is not suppressed by the POP (unlike the combined pill). Levonorgestrel does not transfer to the milk unlike norethisterone which has a plasma: milk ratio of 10:1. Lactation has a contraceptive effect making potent methods like the COC pill less necessary (see 'the lactational amenorrhoea method' under 'Natural family planning')

- **Menopause**: the timing of the menopause will be unaffected by the POP. Unlike the COC pill the POP will not mask the menopause and so menstrual irregularity, amenorrhoea and climacteric symptoms due to oestrogen deficiency may occur. In addition, the problem of functional ovarian cysts may be increased

- **Menstrual pattern** is unaffected in just under half of all women using the POP. In some amenorrhoea develops (see above) and in the remaining women erratic menstruation is the rule. Although erratic menstruation is far from ideal it is associated with a lower failure rate than regular menstruation. Specific counselling on this issue is essential before a woman starts the POP. If it is totally unexpected it will probably be intolerable

- **Migraine** is a relative contraindication (absolute if severe or complicated) to the COC pill but not the POP. Migraine sufferers can use the POP although women with focal or severe disease should be observed carefully

- **Missed or late pills** constitute the biggest cause of POP contraceptive failure. One of the contraceptive actions of the POP (especially in women whose menstrual pattern is unchanged when using the POP) is on cervical mucus. The effect takes four hours to develop, decreases around 22 hours after the last dose and disappears by 36 hours. Professor Guillebaud (1994) advises extra precautions if a woman is more than three hours late in taking her pill and these precautions should continue for the following seven days. If unprotected intercourse has taken place within the previous 72 hours, emergency contraception should be given. For legal reasons the drug manufacturers state 14 days of added precautions should be taken. Women who find difficulty taking pills regularly are not ideal candidates for the POP ('Timing'; see below)

- **Osteoporosis** is not prevented by the POP. In fact, women who are rendered amenorrhoeic may be at marginally greater risk. Guillebaud (1994) suggests that women using the POP in whom amenorrhoea occurs should, after five years, have a serum oestradiol assay and a bone scan to see if a significant hypo-oestrogenic state has developed. In such women, alternative contraceptive measures or add-back oestrogens can be considered

- **Ovarian cysts** related to the function of the ovary (ie. not neoplastic) are not infrequent in POP users. Many are asymptomatic and only diagnosed if an ultrasound scan happens to be done. They can cause pain which may be severe enough to mimic ectopic pregnancy. They may be more common in older POP users (Guillebaud, 1994)

- **Sickle cell disease** is characterised by thrombotic crises. Pregnancy is hazardous. The oestrogen-free methods are particularly beneficial and depot medroxyprogesterone acetate has been shown to provide excellent contraception as well as reducing the incidence of crises. The POP is also suitable for women with sickle cell disease

- **Smokers**: the POP is not contraindicated in smokers, even those over 35 years of age

- **Teenage contraception**: precision in time of taking is critical with the POP. Although an effective method, it is less strongly indicated in highly fertile young women. Non-barrier methods also have particular drawbacks in younger women. These relate to reliability of taking the pill regularly and exposure to seminal fluid.

    Seminal fluid, in addition to carrying the risk of pregnancy, can also carry sexually transmitted diseases. These may be more likely in women who are not in monogamous stable relationships. The juvenile cervix which may not have completed its squamous metaplasia is vulnerable to neoplastic influences. To protect against this and STD young women using oral contraception are advised to employ a barrier method (usually condoms) in addition to oral contraception

- **Thromboembolic disease** is not exacerbated in POP users. The POP can be used in women with a past (but not active or current) history of venous thromboembolic disorder

- **Timing** is crucial in using the POP. Cervical mucus effects take four hours to develop after taking each pill and decline from around 22 hours. Delaying more than three hours after the time which the next dose is due to be taken, compromises contraceptive efficacy, especially in women with regular periods when using the POP. Some account must be taken of the most likely times intercourse takes place in order to work out when each day's pill should be taken (see 'Missed or late pills', above).

Levonorgestrel intrauterine system LNG-IUS

The range of contraceptive options available to women today is wider than ever before. These options divide roughly into barrier methods, intrauterine devices and hormonal contraceptives. One can also add natural family planning, spermicides and sterilisation to this list. Recently, a new method has become available to women in the United Kingdom; the levonorgestrel intrauterine system (IUS). This device is a hybrid whose antecedents are hormonal contraceptives and intrauterine devices. See *Box 3.7* and *Tables 3.5* and *3.6*.

Box 3.7: The levonorgestrel intrauterine system

Mirena the LNG-IUS
Indications: Contraception (possibly menorrhagia and progesterone opposition to oestrogen HRT in the future)
Cautions: Depression, liver dysfunction, diseases prone to worsen in pregnancy, diabetes, hypertension
Contraindications: Pregnancy or suspected pregnancy, undiagnosed vaginal bleeding, uterine anomaly, genital infection, PID, severe arterial disease, haematological malignancy, recent trophoblastic disease, acute or severe liver disease, immunodeficiency
Interactions: Liver enzyme inducing drugs, ie. carbamazepine, phenylbutazone, barbiturates, phenytoin, primidone, griseofulvin and rifampicin are listed in MIMS

NB. Mirena is not licensed for post coital/emergency contraception

Table 3.5: Depot progestins including Norplant and Mirena

Product	Dose	Presentation	Progestin class	Duration of efficacy	Cost per dose £	Cost per annum £
Depo-Provera medroxyprogesterone acetate	150 mg/ml 1ml im	aqueous suspension	pregnane	12 weeks	4.55	19.72
Implanon etonogestrel	68 mg single implant	1 x silastic rod	gonane	3 years	90	30(x3)
Noristerat norethisterone enanthate	200 mg/ml 1 ml im	oily suspension	gonane	8 weeks	3.00	19.50
Mirena levonorgestrel	52 mg (20 mcg/24 hours)	progestin in silastic sleeve on 'T'-shaped IUD	gonane	5 years *	89.25	19.85 (x5)

Principal sources: *MIMS*, November 1999; *BNF* **38**, September 1999

Notes:
* Probable effective life more than five years, current licence for three years only
x5 Cost of method if used over three or five years respectively
pregnane   progesterone derived
gonane   testosterone derived

The intrauterine element of the IUS is a plastic 'T'-shaped scaffold. The Mirena IUS, the only device on the market at present, is identical to the Nova T IUD without its copper attachments. The hormonal element is the progestogen levonorgestrel which is attached to the vertical shaft of the plastic intrauterine device as a collar reservoir of hormone enclosed in a slow release membrane. The contraceptive effects of the IUS are the result of the action of levonorgestrel directly on the endometrium. You could describe the IUS as a 'laser targeted minipill' in that it is a progestogen only contraceptive, which acts precisely on the end organ with minimal collateral systemic effects. The dose released is 20 mcg/24 hour, producing a serum level of around one quarter that of the oral POP.

The IUS has been described by leading authorities in this country as a breakthrough in contraceptive provision and initial enthusiasm has not waned since its UK launch in July 1995. The reasons for this enthusiasm are several. Firstly, it provides reversible contraception which relies neither on user action around the time of intercourse nor on a daily routine of pill-taking. It is highly effective, with failure rates lower than those seen with the combined oral contraceptive pill and even sterilisation. Its duration of action is five years. The extension of its licensed lifespan from three to five years was conferred retrospectively on Mirenas already *in situ*. Its principal non-contraceptive benefit, however, is that in thinning the endometrium it reduces the amount of tissue that can be shed at the time of menstruation. After several months of use the total menstrual blood loss per cycle drops dramatically, so much so that some women will cease having any show during their menstrual phase. This effect is purely on the end organ of female fertility, the endometrium. The systemic effects are rarely more than minimal. Small wonder therefore that much interest has been shown by women and their attendants.

There are two difficulties that have to be faced before embarking on providing a IUS fitting service:

- Firstly, the IUS is not cheap. It costs around £90 per device although, being a contraceptive, it is provided free of charge to the women wishing it to be fitted. This cost is up-front money and if divided by its duration of action, five years, then the cost per month of use is not very different from other forms of contraception. This calculation takes no account of its non-contraceptive benefits which in the case of a menorrhagic woman, contemplating hysterectomy, are not inconsiderable

- Secondly, the straw that is used to place the device into the uterus is wider than most other IUDs with an external diameter of 4.8 mm. This is because the collar of the levonorgestrel is attached around the vertical shaft. The consequence is that some women require cervical dilation to enable comfortable and easy placement of the device. The cervix can be dilated with graded sounds but some form of analgesia is necessary for this to be done

Table 3.6: IUDs

Device	Active component	licensed lifespan (years)	probable lifespan (years) *	fail rate per HWY
Multiload Cu 250 and Cu 250 Short	Cu	3	3	1–2
Multiload Cu 250 (short)	Cu	3	3	1–2
Multiload Cu 375 **	Cu	5	8	2.9 @ 5years
Nova T	Ag/Cu	5	3	5.5 @ 5 years
Nova T 380**	Ag/Cu	5	5	1.4 @ 5 years
Gynae T 380 slimline ** d/c from 1/2000	Cu	8	8	1.7 @ 3 years
GyneFix	Cu	5	5	0.5 @ 3 years
Flexi-T	Cu	data awaited		0.6 @ 1 year
(Mirena)	LNG	5	5	0.4 @ 5 years

Notes:
*	In women over 40 years, newly fitted IUDs may be left in situ until after the menopause (Tacchi D, 1990)
**	3° generation Cu devices
Cu	copper
Ag	silver
LNG	levonorgestrel
HWY	hundred women years

Inert devices are no longer marketed although some women may still have one *in utero*

NB: Although it was formerly stated that 'no copper IUD needs replacing routinely in less than five years' (ref DTB 1990, 28: 11–12) a recent communication recommends that IUDs with low surface areas, ie. 250mm2 should not be relied upon after three years of use and state the 'choice if a copper T Cu 380A or a Copper T Cu 380 slimline is not available, would appear to be between the GyneFix, Mirena IUS, Multiload MLCu 375, or Nova T 380' (FFP Faculty News, November, 1999).

Suitability

The IUS is a suitable form of contraception for women requiring long term, reversible control of fertility. It is easier to say for whom the system would not be suitable. This group would include:

- **women known to be or suspected of being pregnant:** **NB**: the IUS is not licensed for emergency contraception

- **women with very small uteri** that may not accommodate the full length of the device

- **women with a distorted uterus**, fibroids being the commonest cause although not all fibroids will enlarge or distort the uterine lumen

- **women with active pelvic infection** is an obvious contraindication. A past history is a less strong contraindication and may in fact be less likely in IUS users. The IUS protected uterus may be hostile to infection as well as pregnancy

- **women with genital tract malignancy** including trophoblastic disease

- **women with ethical objections** to the method may decline the LNG-IUS for the same reasons as they would decline the IUD or the progestogen only pill; all three methods will occasionally result in the failure of an embryo to implant. The manufacturers advise consideration of termination of breakthrough pregnancies with an IUS *in situ*. For some women this may be enough of a reason to decline using this method

- **pre-menarche and postmenopausal women**

- **women with cardiac defects** where there may be a risk of endocarditis

- **women with immunodeficiency**: HIV seropositivity is a contraindication to all forms of IUD

- **women with diabetes mellitus and prior ectopic pregnancy** are relative contraindications.

Counselling/workup

No matter how good a method of contraception is there will always be the possibility of unwanted effects. Counselling women involves informing them of the potential drawbacks as well as the expected benefits. Only then can an informed choice be made. If a problem arises after fitting the device, eg. vaginal spotting, the woman who knows it was a possibility but chose the method nevertheless, will usually be tolerant. The uninformed woman may well be angry and dissatisfied. The particular points that must be covered for those considering having an IUS fitted are:

- **how the IUS works**: the principal effects are on the endometrium which decidualises and thins rendering it hostile to sperm and embryos. The IUS also affects cervical mucus and tubal secretions. There will be variable effects on ovulation with occasional anovulatory cycles

- **expulsion rates** are low (2–5%) but as with IUD are clustered in the first few weeks after fitting. Continuation of existing or alternative contraceptive methods, for the IUS first cycle at least, is recommended followed by a check-up to ensure that the device is still in place before full reliance on the IUS for contraception

- **failure rates** are low. Very occasional failure has been reported (around one per 500 woman years of use)

- **menstrual pattern change** is the rule. Erratic bleeding or vaginal spotting occurs for up to four months in some women. Occasionally the problem persists. Most women will settle down to a regular cycle which then becomes lighter and shorter month by month. By one year up to 20% of women will be rendered amenorrhoeic, despite a regular ovarian 'menstrual' cycle. The message that women should take away is that their hormonal cycles will carry on but there will be so little womb lining that a show of blood may not occur despite their being in the menstrual phase of a normal cycle

- **progestational side-effects** are possible but uncommon. Blood levels from the LNG-IUS are around one quarter of those using LNG minipills. It is, however, possible for premenstrual type symptoms to develop as well as breast symptoms of swelling and mastalgia and skin changes like acne to occur

- **insertion and removal technique** should be covered and are discussed in detail below

- **cervical anaesthesia and dilation** is a particular requirement for many women opting for this device. This is discussed in more detail below.

How to fit the LNG-IUS

The manufacturers of the 'Mirena' IUS state in their prescribing information that their device should be fitted only by a health professional who has received practical training, such as that provided by the Faculty of Family Planning of the Royal College of Obstetricians and Gynaecologists. Fitting is the same as with an IUD except that cervical dilation and paracervical anaesthesia are perhaps a little more likely to be required. The key steps in fitting an IUS are as follows:

- *only do easy insertions*: uterine penetration and perforation are more likely if force is used. Uterine position and cervical canal tone vary with the time in the menstrual cycle. If difficulties are encountered consider abandoning the procedure and trying again another day

- *vaginal and endocervical microbiological swabs* should be taken. These should be taken prior to insertion. By identifying and treating women with pathogens it will be possible to reduce the incidence of post-fitting sepsis by giving early treatment. Vaginal swabs for bacterial vaginosis and endocervical swabs for chlamydia trachomatis are advisable

- *pregnancy* should be excluded either by fitting the IUS during the menstrual phase, or if fitting is done later in the cycle either by continuing excellent contraception or abstinence from sexual relations

- *local anaesthesia* may be required for comfortable insertion of the device. Injecting 0.5–1 ml of local anaesthetic at the 12 o'clock position where the tenaculum will be attached is kind. Instillation of anaesthetic gel along the cervical canal will reduce discomfort but the effect is said to be small and there is a theoretical risk of microbial contamination of the upper cervical canal and uterus. Lignocaine 2% gel (Instillagel) can be used. The alternative method is to administer a para-cervical block. This is discussed below

- *a significant analgesic effect* will also be obtained by pre-medicating the woman with a non-steroidal anti-inflammatory drug. Unless there are contraindications to their use (peptic ulceration, asthma) Ibuprofen 400–600 mg with food one hour prior to insertion will give reasonable analgesia. Because of their anti-prostaglandin activities NSAIDs will also reduce post insertion cramps and, it is said, the expulsion rate. Some operators advise taking NSAIDs for a day or two after insertion to maximise this effect

- *sounding the endocervical canal and uterus* is vital in all IUD/IUS placements as is a preliminary pelvic examination to assess uterine size and position

- *dilation of the endocervical canal and endocervical os* is frequently required in order that the slightly broader IUS fitting straw be passed with ease. Familiarity with cervical dilation is required and this should be covered in training for IUD fitting. Sounding should only follow after the uterine size and position has been established. This allows the uterine and, to a degree, the cervical component of its length to be established. If a 5 mm sound passes the internal os then passage of the IUS should be simple. Dilate the internal cervical os beginning with the largest sound you estimate will pass easily. Idilate to 5 mm. Use of dilators requires adequate training

- *management of collapse*: vasovagal stimulation during IUD/IUS fitting is not uncommon. It is rare that anything other than the head down position and leg elevation will be needed. Occasionally, a profound bradycardia may require the administration of atropine. Asystole and the need for adrenaline is a rarity but an 'in date' resuscitation tray should always be available at IUD/IUS fitting sessions. Oxygen, intravenous lines and intubation equipment are ideal.

para-cervical block

The more fit LNG-IUSs I have fitted, the less I have to resort to paracervical block. It is now a very occasional requirement in my practice. The sensory nerve supply to the cervix is mainly via the uterosacral ligaments. These insert into the cervix at the 4 and 8 o'clock positions when the cervix is viewed in the lithotomy position. The following routine may be followed:

- ensure that you are assisted by a competent nurse. A good assistant provides at least half of the analgesic effect

- draw up 10 ml of 0.5% xylocaine in a 10 ml syringe with a green 21F needle attached

- inject 0.5 ml of anaesthetic at 12 o'clock where the tenaculum will be applied and 0.5 ml at 4 and 8 o'clock into the cervix to numb the skin where the main injections will be given

- attach a single toothed tenaculum at 12 o'clock and apply traction to straighten the path into the uterus and stabilise it

- inject the remaining anaesthetic liquid, 4–5 ml on either side. The point of injection should be placed two thirds of the distance from the edge of the os to the lateral cervical wall. The green 21F needle should be inserted to its hub parallel to the cervical canal and the anaesthetic instilled mostly at the level of the internal os with the remainder injected as the needle is withdrawn. Countertraction with a tenaculum is required. The nurse will have to discreetly feed back how the woman is coping as it is impossible to inject and watch the woman's face at the same time

- do not be alarmed at the bleeding that follows injections in the cervix; although sometimes dramatic looking it is in fact trivial and abates spontaneously within seconds. Usual losses are around 10–20 mls

- horizontal rest and observation of the patient after insertion

- paracervical analgesia takes around five minutes to develop.

Follow up

If any problems develop in the first few days after insertion the women should have *carte blanche* for a return consultation. Most will have no problems and will be seen after the next period to ensure that the device has not been expelled and to be advised that the IUS can be used as the sole contraceptive method. Encouraging women to check their own threads by vaginal examination after each period is strongly advisable. In oligoamenorrhoeic women (eg. postpartum) advise a one month check for the same purpose. Also ask them to return after their next period for review. Once the device is *in situ* an annual check up is all that is required unless problems or questions arise. The levonorgestel IUS generally gives excellent low-maintenance contraception.

Non-contraceptive benefits of Mirena

- menstrual blood loss is dramatically reduced

- dysmenorrhoea is usually greatly reduced

- iron deficiency as a consequence is reduced

- uterine fibroids at least are less likely to grow and may indeed shrink

- pelvic infection is uncommon, there may be a protective effect in IUS wearers

- endometrial hyperplasia and atypia are prevented and in established cases appear to reverse

- hormonal replacement may be an indication in the future. The LNG-IUS could be used to provide the progestogen in systemic oestrogen HRT users.

Complications of Mirena

- trauma as with any IUD fitting

- failure of contraception is rare. Insertion in early pregnancy must be avoided and early expulsion must be actively checked for

- pelvic infection is rare, especially if vaginal and endocervical swabs taken prior to insertion are negative

- ectopic pregnancy rates may be reduced, a previous ectopic is considered a relative contraindication

- progestational side-effects are possible but far fewer than with oral progestogens and probably less than with Norplant

- erratic vaginal blood loss is very common in the first two or three months after fitting. It rarely persists

- oligoamenorrhoea may be considered a side-effect if counselling has been incomplete

- functional ovarian cysts are a recognised complication of oral progestogen contraceptives. Similar functional cyst formation may occur with the IUS but the likelihood of clinical significance is considered minimal.

Depot progestogens

See *Table 3.5*. Parenteral progestogens come in three main forms:

- **depot injections** See *Box 3.8*
- **implants** See *Box 3.9*
- **the levonorgestrel intrauterine system** (discussed above)

Depot injections

See *Box 3.8* and *Table 3.5*. Long term depot progestogens provide contraception by suppressing ovulation as well as having contraceptive effects on the endometrium and cervical mucus. Some follicular activity does occur and as a result oestrogen deficiency is rarely a problem. They are highly effective and convenient contraceptives with numerous beneficial side-effects (eg. reduced anaemia, dysmenorrhoea, PID, ectopic gestation, endometrial cancer). Depot progestogens are particularly suited to women who are prone to forgetting or being late for oral methods. They do not require action at the time of intercourse and in the case of Depo-Provera require just four attendances per year to maintain contraceptive cover. Women with physical disability may find depot methods very suitable as dexterity is not required and the amenorrhoea which often ultimately develops may be welcomed. Depot methods have a long history of use in women with mental disability too, but beware interactions with anti-convulsant drugs.

Box 3.8: Depot injected progestogens

Depo-Provera and Noristerat
Indications: Contraception
Cautions: Depression, liver dysfunction, diseases prone to worsen in pregnancy, diabetes, undiagnosed vaginal bleeding
Contraindications: Pregnancy or suspected pregnancy, hormone dependent cancer including current or recent trophoblastic disease, acute or severe liver disease, previous pregnancy-associated pemphigoid gestationis, pruritis or jaundice, thromboembolic disease
Interactions: Enzyme inducing drugs, ie. carbamazepine, phenylbutazone, barbiturates, phenytoin, primidone, griseofulvin, rifampicin

NB: Depot methods are licensed as 'second choice' methods to be used only after counselling. They are, however, first rate methods and are under-used in the UK

Drawbacks of the method principally include:

- ***menstrual cycle disturbance*** which after an unpredictable initial phase usually settles down to produce amenorrhoea
- ***weight gain*** often occurs and may be as much as 4–5 lb. It may be commoner in slim women
- ***fertility*** return is slower than with oral methods and this may be a deciding factor in some women. The slope and shape of the cumulative conception rate curves parallels that of women using other methods, but is shifted to the right by about five months from the time of the last injection when compared with methods that reverse more rapidly
- ***less frequent side-effects*** include tiredness, low mood, lower libido, mastalgia

- **osteoporosis** has been suggested to be a risk. The studies suggesting this are small and open to criticism and against them must be weighed the total lack of clinical evidence of osteoporotic fractures in long term users. It is something to be considered and for this reason depot progestogens are not recommended in women approaching the menopause. As with amenorrhoea on the POP, five years of amenorrhoea should prompt screening for hypo-oestrogenism by taking a serum oestradiol level and arranging a bone scan (Guillebaud, 1994)

Product differences

Depo-Provera has a longer and more world-wide pedigree. Noristerat is used more frequently in Germany. Depo-Provera is an aqueous solution which is injected twelve-weekly unlike Noristerat which is oily and requires an eight-weekly injection. Noristerat is licensed for short term use and may be indicated where reversibility of a depot method is preferred. Once-a-month formulations may be available in the near future. Depo-Provera is a pregnane (progesterone derived) progestogen. Noristerat is a gonane (testosterone derived).

Depot injected progestogens: key issues

- **Age**: women over 45 years are unsuited to depot injections as they may add to their osteoporotic risk by enhancing the reduced oestrogenic effects of the climacteric
- **Breast cancer** is almost certainly not caused/increased by use of depot progestogens. High doses of medroxyprogesterone acetate have been linked to breast cancer in beagle bitches, but it has now been shown that this breed of dog has an inherent susceptibility to breast tumours and is an inappropriate comparison species
- **Cancer risks** are either unaffected or in the case of the endometrium are reduced in women using depot progestogens. Use of depot progestogens should be deferred until hCG levels are normal in cases of trophoblastic disease
- **Commencement of depot injections** in regularly cycling women should be before day five and if possible (to guarantee immediate contraception) on day one or two of the cycle. Women on the COC or POP who are not pregnant can have a depot injection at any time. Contraception at times other than days one or two may not be immediate; extra precautions needed for one week
- **Coronary artery disease** risks are unaffected. There are suggestions that reduced oestrogen levels which can result from long term depot progestogen contraception can reduce HDL-cholesterol and this could enhance atheroma formation
- **Ectopic pregnancy** risks are reduced as ovulation is prevented
- **Endometriosis** is probably reduced as are PID and functional ovarian cysts
- **Epilepsy** is not a contraindication to depot progestogens. However, enzyme inducing anti-convulsants can accelerate progestogen metabolism. Family planning consultants often advise reducing the interval between injection in such circumstances
- **Fertility returns**, as mentioned above, about five months after the last injection of Depo-Provera. Long term fertility is unaffected
- **Hypertension** is not caused by depot progestogens and is not a contraindication
- **Menopause** may be masked because of amenorrhoea by depot progestogens. Depot progestogens are not recommended in women over 45 years. Premature menopause could be partially masked by depot progestogens
- **Overdue injections** pose a risk of contraceptive failure. It is generally thought that seven days of leeway exist, so contraceptive cover continues to the end of the ninth week for

Noristerat and to the end of the thirteenth week since the last injection for Depo-Provera. Delays later than that should be followed by emergency contraceptive advice and provision if indicated. Recommencement of depot contraception requires a negative pregnancy test if intercourse has occurred

- **Post-abortal use**: depot injections are usually given on the seventh day following abortion or miscarriage. For late abortions/miscarriages delaying further should be considered as the situation becomes analogous to postpartum use (see below)

- **Postpartum use** should be deferred until six weeks after delivery, irrespective of lactation. Use earlier than this can cause heavy vaginal bleeding

- **Sickle cell disease** (homozygous SS and SC) is probably ameliorated in women using Depo-Provera, which is therefore the usual first choice contraceptive method in affected women

- **Surgery** is not a contraindication to depot methods as they do not promote thromboembolic disorder. They are in fact a useful method in women wanting contraception and facing surgery

- **Teratogenesis** has been suggested but not proved. Masculinisation of a female fetus and external genital anomalies in male fetuses (hypospadias) have been reported but their significance is disputed

- **Thromboembolic disease** is not affected by depot progestogens which can therefore be given to women with a past (but not active or current) thromboembolic disorder.

Progestogen implants

See *Box 3.9* and *Table 3.5*. Progestogen implants are available as 'Norplant', a six rod levonorgestrel implant system providing five years of continuous contraception after which the rods have to be removed. A trochar is used to place the rods in a fan array under the skin on the inner aspect of the upper arm. This requires training. Removal can be quite difficult and also requires training. A single rod system will be launched in 1999 (Implanon — for a review see *Br J Fam Planning*, 1999, **24**: supplement).

Box 3.9: The levonorgestrel implant

Norplant: the LNG implant
Indications: Contraception
Cautions: Hypertension, arterial disease risk, benign intracranial hypertension, migraine
Contraindications: Pregnancy or suspected pregnancy, severe arterial disease, thromboembolic disorder, risk of severe ischaemic heart disease, undiagnosed vaginal bleeding, hormone dependent cancer including recent trophoblastic disease, acute or severe liver disease
Interactions: Carbamazepine, phenylbutazone, barbiturates, phenytoin, primidone, griseofulvin, rifampicin

A certificate of approved experience, granted after training approved by a college, is now required for Norplant fitting. For details contact: The Faculty of Family Planning and Reproductive Health Care of The Royal College of Obstetricians and Gynaecologists. If there is any room left on the envelope you can add the address which is 27 Sussex Place, Regents Park, London NW1 4RG.

LNG-implants: key issues:

- **Arterial disease** is a relative contraindication. Manufacturers recommend removal of rods if arterial disease occurs in women fitted with Norplant

- **Benign intracranial hypertension** has been reported in Norplant users. Women developing significant headaches or visual problems should be checked for BIH. A less informative synonym for BIH which is used in North America is pseudotumor cerebri

- **Commencement regimes**: in regularly menstruating women fitting on day one of the cycle gives immediate contraception. Between days 2–5 fitting should be followed by additional precautions for a further week. Fitting later in the cycle requires that pregnancy is excluded and additional measures taken for seven days

  After childbirth, Norplant can be inserted on day 21. If fitted later than this additional measures are required for seven days. Small quantities of levonorgestrel will enter the milk. After abortion, Norplant can be inserted immediately. Insertion after day 5 should be followed by additional precautions for seven days

- **Ectopic pregnancy** is reduced compared with non-contracepting women. The greater reduction in intrauterine pregnancy makes the ratio of breakthrough pregnancies being ectopic higher than among non-contraceptors. This is similar to that seen in Mirena and POP

- **Fertility return** is rapid after Norplant removal: *circa* 2 days

- **Functional ovarian cysts** are uncommon but can occur and as with POP can cause symptoms. However, abdominal pain should always prompt exclusion of ectopic pregnancy

- **Hypertension** is not a contraindication and only a rare complication of Norplant

- **Menstrual pattern** can change with Norplant and women must be counselled about this before fitting. Polymenorrhoea is the commonest reason for premature removal of Norplant (around 10% by 12 months). It tends to settle over time. Amenorrhoea can occur too. If it follows regular menstruation on Norplant pregnancy should be excluded

- **Migraine** is uncommon, but new, deteriorating, focal or crescendo migraine should prompt removal of Norplant. Consider benign intracranial hypertension for persistent headache

- **Pregnancy** should be excluded as described above under commencement regimes. If pregnancy should occur with Norplant in situ, the rods should be removed

- **Side-effects** most commonly include menstrual pattern change and amenorrhoea. Acne has been described, as has weight changes, nausea, mastalgia and breast discharge, hair changes (hypertrichosis and scalp hair loss), mood changes, cervicitis and vaginitis

- **Surgery** is not a reason to remove Norplant. Usual anti-thrombotic measures should be applied if major surgery is undertaken

- **Thromboembolism**, if active and current, is a contraindication. A previous history is a relative contraindication of the method although the manufacturers advise that it can be used if a risk: benefit assessment suggests it is preferred.

Intrauterine contraceptive devices

See *Box 3.10*. The intrauterine contraceptive devices (IUD) are all copper bearing with the exception of the levonorgestrel intrauterine system (LNG-IUS, Mirena). Details of the IUDs are listed in *Table 3.6*.

Box 3.10: The intrauterine contraceptive device

Indications: Reversible long term contraception, emergency contraception

Cautions: Nulliparity, youth, previous ectopic gestation (in nulliparous women contraindication), possible subfertility, lifestyle risk of sexually transmitted disease, primary dysmenorrhoea, endometriosis, menorrhagia, uterine fibroids, congenital uterine anomaly, scarred uterus, cervical stenosis, prior endometrial ablation/resection, previous pelvic sepsis, valvular heart disease, prior prosthetic surgery, corticosteroid therapy

Contraindications: Irregular or undiagnosed genital tract bleeding, genital tract malignancy, acute or chronic pelvic infection, previous ectopic gestation in nulliparous women, suspicion of pregnancy, dyspareunia, recent possible exposure to sexually transmitted disease (eg. rape), previous tubal surgery, distorted uterine cavity, previous bacterial endocarditis, prosthetic heart valve, anatomical heart lesion, immunosuppressive therapy, HIV/AIDS, allergy to constituents, Wilson's disease (for copper devices)

Interactions: pencillamine

Details on cervical block anaesthesia are discussed above in the LNG-IUS section. The pros and cons of the IUDs are listed in *Box 3.11*.

Box 3.11: Pros and cons of IUDs

Advantages	Disadvantages/complications
• very effective contraception	• heavier menstrual blood loss *
• reversible contraception	• dysmenorrhoea increased *
• contraception independent of coitus	• exacerbated intercurrent genital infection
• no daily routine to be forgotten	• pelvic actinomycosis risk
• inexpensive *	• uterine malposition/penetration/perforation
• lactation unaffected	• pregnancy (method failure)
• defers sterilisation	• post fitting infection and expulsion
• no systemic side-effects *	• miscarriage risk in breakthrough pregnancies

*with the exception of the LNG-IUS

Key issues

- **Actinomycosis**: the detection of the bacterium *actinomycosis Israeli* is commoner in women who carry an IUD than in women who do not. Asymptomatic detection is usually made during cervical cytological analysis. The organism which may be a commensal but suppurative pelvic actinomycosis has been described in the literature. The incidence in women with IUDs is extremely low. Current advice is that the presence of the organism in a woman without symptoms does not require the removal of the IUD. If the woman is happy to continue using her IUD and to have regular pelvic examination to exclude the development of signs of pelvic infection, then the device can be left in situ. Examinations should be performed at least annually. Microbiological analysis of removed IUDs is no longer considered of value.

- **Age** is a significant factor in IUD use. The device, as with other forms of contraception, will be less effective in preventing pregnancy in younger more fertile women. Younger women have a higher chance of acquiring sexually transmitted disease which will be exacerbated in the presence of an IUD. Young women, especially if nulliparous, tend to have smaller uteri and therefore a higher chance of fitting difficulties and expulsion. The choice in younger women with small uteri is between the Nova T and the Multiload Cu 250 (short) although this device may require a paracervical block for fitting (Guillebaud, 1994).

Older women, on the other hand (>40 years), can keep a newly-fitted copper IUD until after the menopause, as fecundity wanes rapidly and coil change will only increase the risk of contraceptive failure

- **Anaemia** is more common in long term IUD users, with the exception of the LNG-IUS (Mirena)

- **Anaesthesia** is occasionally useful when inserting an IUD. Instillation of anaesthetic gel up the cervical canal may give some benefit but theoretically carries the risk of introduction of vaginal organisms into the uterus. Lignocaine gel 2% (Instillagel) is marketed for use during cervical manipulative procedures. The paracervical block is described above in the section on the LNG-IUS (Mirena)

- **Commencement and removal regimes**: initial fitting in regularly cycling women can be done from any time after the end of the main menstrual flow up until day 19 (ovulation plus five days) if the woman has a 28 day cycle (add a day for each day longer her cycle is). If no intercourse has occurred than it can be fitted after day 19 until the next period appears.

   Post-abortal fitting can be performed immediately but infection can develop in the presence of retained products. Postpartum fitting is usually delayed until six weeks have elapsed. There is no interference with lactation. Care must be taken as the postpartum uterus is more susceptible to penetration and perforation.

   Removal of devices should be preceded by seven days of either avoidance of intercourse or the use of other precautions. The principal effects of the copper IUDs are in the last week of the menstrual cycle. Removal before this time can allow fertilisation and implantation to occur. This advice is especially relevant to women listed for sterilisation. Ideally, devices should not be removed after day 19 of a 28 day cycle

- **Diabetes mellitus** is a relative contraindication to the IUDs because of the slight infection risk associated with both. If infection risk is assumed to be low the IUD can be considered

- **Dyspareunia** is considered a contraindication to the IUD as it may imply infection or endometriosis. Dyspareunia developing after IUD fitting could signify perforation, penetration, movement of the device, partial expulsion and infection. Male dyspareunia should prompt an examination to exclude partial expulsion. Threads, especially if short can cause male dyspareunia. It is acceptable in this circumstance to cut the threads back so that nothing protrudes through the external cervical os

- **Ectopic pregnancy** is not prevented by IUDs as efficiently as intrauterine pregnancies. The ratio of pregnancies that are ectopic is therefore higher with an IUD than in women who conceive without an IUD, although absolute number is reduced. All IUD pregnancies should be assumed to be ectopic until proved otherwise. Because of the particular hazards of pelvic infection deteriorating in women with IUDs, and the link between genital infection and ectopic gestation, a past history of ectopic gestation is a relative contraindication to the IUD and an absolute contraindication in nulliparous women with a past history of ectopic gestation

- **Emergency contraception**: see section on 'Emergency contraception' below

- **Epilepsy** will not be caused by the IUD, however seizures during IUD fitting have been reported

- **Expulsion** of the IUD can occur at any time and is often unnoticed. Expulsion occurs more commonly in the first few weeks after fitting. The less often an IUD is changed the less the risk of expulsion is. Women should be encouraged to check the threads themselves after each period for reassurance that expulsion has not occurred

- **Failure rates** are lowest with the Multiload Cu 375, Gynae T 380 and Mirena-IUS devices (see *Table 3.6*). Failures generally cluster around the time of fitting or changing of devices. The less frequently IUDs are changed the less failure will occur. Failures of copper IUDs have been associated with high and persistent aspirin ingestion

- **Fibroids** are not of themselves a reason to avoid using the IUD. If, however, they distort or enlarge the uterine cavity the IUD is contraindicated

- **Fitting IUDs**: all IUDs have specific insertion instructions with their packaging. It is a prerequisite that the IUD fitter has had approved training and experience. Pre-fitting patient counselling is mandatory. Strict asepsis is essential and the availability of paracervical analgesia is good practice.

   An emergency tray should be available containing atropine for the occasional profound and prolonged vaso-vagal bradycardia that can be provoked by cervical manipulation, and adrenaline for the rare occurrence of life-threatening bronchospasm. Analgesia, oral sedatives and NSAIDs reduce cramps if given prior to fitting

- **Gynefix device**, or CuFix was launched in 1998. It consists of a thread, knotted at one end, which is embedded into the fundal myometrium. Suspended on the thread are copper bands which provide the contraceptive effect (For a review see *Br J Fam Planning*, 1999 **24**: 149–159)

- **Heart disease**: valvular heart disease is a contraindication to the IUD. The risk of bacterial endocarditis outweighs its benefits. The IUD is similarly contraindicated in women with valve prostheses

- **HIV/AIDS** are contraindications to the IUD because of the risks of serious pelvic infection developing in an immunocompromised state. Prolongation of menstruation may be a factor promoting transmission

- **Infertility** may be caused by the IUD in that infection in its presence tends to be more severe and so more likely to damage the fallopian tubes. This is one reason why IUDs are relatively contraindicated in women who have not had a family and even more so in women who are not in a stable mutually monogamous relationship

- **Lifestyle** is relevant to choice of the IUD. The forgetful woman who finds oral contraception hazardous should consider the IUD. Women who are not in a monogamous relationship and therefore at some increased risk of sexually transmitted disease are not good candidates for the IUD. In this circumstance, if the IUD is used the addition of a barrier method and spermicides which have antimicrobial actions should be considered

- **Lactation** is not a contraindication to the IUD. Lactating women have softer and more easily perforated uteri. Extra care during placement should be employed

- **Lost threads** should always prompt testing to exclude pregnancy. If pregnancy is excluded an attempt should be made to identify whether the IUD has been expelled. An ultrasound or X-Ray examination will identify whether the IUD is *in utero* or even within the abdomen. Abdominal IUDs should be removed; refer to a gynaecologist. Threads that have ascended the cervical canal can be retrieved successfully with a cervical brush (rotate as you withdraw)

- **Medicated IUDs** are ones which incorporate a progestogen. The only one currently available is the LNG-IUS (Mirena)

- **Menstruation** tends to become heavier in women using copper IUDs. Prolonged use increases the risk of iron deficiency anaemia. In menorrhagic women copper IUDs are relatively contraindicated. Increased menstrual blood loss has to be discussed with women considering the pill. Some will find this detrimental effect outweighed by positive aspects.

    The LNG-IUS (Mirena) differs from the copper IUDs in that menstrual blood loss decreases and in a proportion of women will stop; ie. the menstrual cycle continues but no endometrium is shed

- **Menopause**: devices should be removed around six months after the apparent final menstrual period. Delay allows involution and cervical stenosis to make removal difficult. Simple contraception measures need to be used until 12–24 months amenorrhoea have passed (see *Chapter 2*)

- **Pelvic infection**, either suspected, active or chronic is a contraindication to the IUD. With the exception of actinomycosis the IUD appears to render any subsequently acquired infections more serious rather than actually causing them in them first place. Most authorities recommend screening for sexually transmissible disease prior to insertion. Screening for chlamydia appears especially important

- **Penetration/perforation** are a particular hazard in the puerperium. The most significant association is operator inexperience especially with uterine malpositions, eg. retroversion. In many cases penetration will only be revealed when pregnancy occurs. Abdominal IUDs should be removed. Previous penetration is not an absolute contraindication to future use of the IUD

- **Pregnancy** can occur with the IUD *in utero*. It is safer to remove the device if the threads are accessible and if it will come gently. Removal is a risk, non-removal is a bigger risk. If the threads are not visible exclude ectopic pregnancy. If the IUD will not come with gentle traction refer to a gynaecologist

- **Tampon use** is generally discouraged immediately after IUD fitting in case the threads should become adherent to the tampon and expulsion be promoted. In established IUD use tampons are not contraindicated as long as they are not left in for too long (12 hours max) and that thread checking is done by the woman after each menstruation

- **Teratogenesis** has not been reported with copper IUDs. Data on teratogenicity with the levonorgestrel IUS (Mirena) is not available

- **Vaginal discharge** can be a sign of infection. A heavier than normal vaginal secretion is not uncommon in women with an IUD

Barrier methods of contraception

See *Tables 3.7* and *3.8*. Female barriers are popular as non-hormonal methods of contraception which are controlled by the woman. Diaphragms work partially as barriers but perhaps principally as reservoirs for spermicides. Caps work as a true barrier but should still be used with spermicides. Caps tend to be prescribed by specialists in family planning whereas diaphragms are commonly prescribed and fitted in the general practice setting as well as the family planning clinic.

Table 3.7: Diaphragms and caps

Device	Varieties	Indication	Sizes
Diaphragms	Type A) (flat spring)	made by Lamberts. No longer NHS prescribable (blacklisted)	55–95 mm 5 mm steps)
	Type B) coiled spring	softer, better in 'sensitive' women or if vaginal muscles are strong	55–95 mm (5 mm steps)
	Type C) all-flex arcing spring	where vaginal walls are lax or cervical position interferes with fitting flat/coiled spring	55–95 mm (5 mm steps)
Caps Cervical cap	Type B — Prentif cavity-rim cap	where diaphragm unsuited. Requires a non-conical, axial cervix	23–31 mm (3 mm steps)
Vault cap	Type A — Dumas	unsuitability of cervical cap or diaphragm	55–75 mm (5 mm steps)
	Type C — Vimule	for the very long cervix; can cause abrasions	42, 48 and 54mm
Condoms	female/male	see text	single size
(Sponge)		(combined barrier spermicide for couples with low fertility)	discontinued sadly (single size)

Diaphragms

Female barrier methods have a very long history. The devices currently available are in essence vehicles for carrying spermicides as well as providing a degree of occlusion against the passage of sperm from the hostile vaginal environment into the friendly cervical canal.

Diaphragms stay in place because of the tension of the metal spring in the rim. Correct choice of size is essential and insertion needs to be taught by an experienced attendant. It is usual for a woman to attend for a check up after prescription of a barrier, with it in place, so that her technique can be assessed.

Spermicidal creams, gels or foams need to be applied to each side of the diaphragm as well as around the rim. Diaphragms can be inserted several hours before intercourse. Extra spermicide should be applied if more than two hours has elapsed. The diaphragm should be removed not less than six hours after the last act of intercourse.

Diaphragms cannot be relied upon to protect against sexually transmitted disease. Although a snug fit may well be found on examination, during intercourse the vagina balloons allowing the diaphragm to move (similar ballooning is sometimes noted during miscarriage).

Contraceptive diaphragms were until recently classified into types A, B and C. The BNF and MIMS now list just two types: the coil spring and the all-flex arcing spring. They correspond to types B and C respectively. MIMS also lists Reflexions, another contraceptive diaphragm made by Lamberts. Sizes range from 55–95 mm rising in 5 mm steps and having a flat spring. They are equivalent to the type A diaphragm but are no longer prescribable on an FP10 (blacklisted).

Caps

Unlike the diaphragm the contraceptive caps are occlusive as well as being reservoirs for spermicides. They rely on suction because of the close application to the vaginal vault or cervix. However, their principal action is as an occlusive barrier and they are not susceptible to the vaginal wall changes during intercourse.

Unlike diaphragms they can be left in place for several days, but 24 hours is the recommended maximum. Prolonged use can lead to malodour. Caps require careful selection of size and expert advice on fitting and use.

Condoms (male)

These are not available on prescription but are available free of charge at family planning clinics and selected general practice outlets. Users should be advised that the condom should be applied to the erect penis before genital contact and penetration. Withdrawal and disposal should be attended to straight after ejaculation ensuring that the condom does not slip off during withdrawal.

Most condoms are manufactured from latex although sheep gut condoms are still available. Latex condoms come with spermicides incorporated into the lubricant. Hypo-allergenic condoms are marketed.

Condoms provide protection against pregnancy and sexually transmitted disease. They reduce the chance of acquiring the HIV infection. There is also evidence that teenage women are more disposed to developing cervical intraepithelial neoplasia if they employ a non-barrier form of contraception. For this reason, as well as for the protection the condom affords against sexually transmitted disease, a barrier should be part of the overall precautions girls and young women use if they decide to engage in full sexual relations.

Caution: Latex can be damaged by a variety of compounds which can lead to a loss of strength and rupture of the sheath. These include baby oils, suntan oils and creams, and many vaginal medications for treatment of fungal infections. Vaseline and petroleum jelly will weaken condoms, but KY-jelly which is aqueous based will not. Certain vaginal topical oestrogens will also damage condoms.

Condom failure, accident or omission should prompt users to seek emergency contraception advice. Additional spermicides are not currently thought to add much to the contraceptive effects of the condom and may, because of the added interference in spontaneity, be counterproductive.

Condom (female)

Available over the counter, the Femidom is a barrier method under the woman's control. It is a lubricated polyurethane sleeve, sealed at one end. A 70 mm ring is incorporated into the external open end. A second smaller ring, to aid insertion in a similar fashion to the contraceptive diaphragm, is located near the upper inner end.

The Femidom is fitted before sexual activity and can remain in place well after ejaculation has occurred. It is a barrier and protects against sexually transmitted disease as well as pregnancy.

At first sight many women find it daunting. It can make a rustling noise during use. One survey reported that men found the Femidom allowed for more sensation than the male condom. Parallel coitus, ie. inside the vagina but outside the Femidom is a hazard to be aware of. The method has not yet taken off. 'Eroginising the condom' has proved difficult in safe sex campaigns; eroginising the Femidom will be a challenge for even the most persuasive of advertising executives, not least because of a failure of primary care professionals to offer it as part of a woman's menu of contraceptive options in the first place.

Spermicidal agents

See *Table 3.8*. Spermicides are generally advised for use as supplements to other methods. Indeed the contraceptive diaphragms are primarily designed to carry spermicides as well as having some action as a barrier. Spermicides have a mild bactericidal action.

Use of spermicides as the sole method of contraception is advisable only in couples with low fertility (eg. perimenopausally, oligospermia) or as a method of family spacing in couples wishing for another child.

Table 3.8: Spermicides

Product	Formulation	Agent	Strength	Pack size
Delfen	foam	Nonoxynol-9	12.5%	20 g Applicator in pack
Double check	pessary	Nonoxynol-9	6%	10 g Applicator in pack
Duragel	gel	Nonoxynol-9	2%	100 g
Gynol II	jelly	Nonoxynol-9	2%	81 g
Ortho-Cream	cream (A)	Nonoxynol-9	2%	70 g
Ortho-Forms	pessary	Nonoxynol-9	5%	15

Principal sources: *MIMS*, November 1999; *BNF* **38**, September 1999

Notes:
(A) applicator available separately
Certain products were previously listed as 'for use as sole method of contraception'. This advice no longer stands.
Spermicides are for use alongside another method, eg. cap, condom, diaphragm

Natural methods of family planning

There is more to natural family planning than the rhythm method. Natural family planning in the UK is an under-used method of child spacing. It has a high failure rate and if pregnancy would be a disaster it is not the method of choice. It requires discipline and commitment. Above all it requires abstinence from penetrative vaginal sexual intercourse at times when libido may be at its peak and fecundity its greatest. For women with moral objections to so-called artificial contraception (ie. when the method as well as the motive is artificial) and for women where other methods are contraindicated then natural family planning is a viable option for the committed enthusiast.

The most effective forms of natural family planning are the lactational amenorrhoea method and the double-check method. The double check relates to the use of techniques to predict both the start and the end of the fertile phase.

For women interested in natural family planning it is essential that they at least read a good text on the subject and are preferably in contact with an experienced instructor. Natural family planning is not a soft option. It requires dedication and meticulous record keeping. In its favour it has to be said that with the exception of unplanned pregnancy there are no side-effects.

The recent introduction of the Persona device is an aid to natural family planning. Very limited trials suggest that it is as effective as other methods of natural family planning. Cervical palpitation and mucus assessment are not required. The system incorporates a kit for testing urine on certain days. The device that analyses the sample has an indicator to tell the woman whether or not sexual intercourse is safe. The device is available over-the-counter from pharmacists.

The options

The rhythm or calendar method

Menstrual records are kept. Over the six most recent cycles the longest and shortest cycles are counted. The beginning day of the fertile phase is calculated as (the shortest cycle length –20 days). The end of the fertile phase is calculated as (the longest cycle –11 days). The time between these dates is regarded as potentially fertile and couples should abstain from intercourse. This method is quite simple in theory although considered to be both unnecessarily restrictive and associated with a high failure rate. As one commentator put it 'Don't knock it. If it wasn't for the rhythm method, I wouldn't have been here today' (Connolly, 1994).

The temperature method

In the late 1930s the sustained rise in basal body temperature (BBT) that begins at the time of ovulation was discovered. The rise is of the order of 0.2°C. A fertility thermometer is needed to measure this (range 29–35°C). A basal temperature is obtained by taking a reading on waking each morning before rising or drinking. Many factors can interfere with the BBT, eg. alcohol, a late night, a lie in (the weekend effect), stress, illness. The temperature method can only detect the end of the fertile phase which comes after the third consecutive day of sustained temperature elevation.

The cervical mucus or 'Billings' method

This relies on the cyclical changes of mucus secreted by the cervical glands. Practitioners of this method inspect their cervical mucus looking at colour, glossiness, fluidity, transparency and stretchiness. They also record their vaginal sensations of dryness, moistness or wetness. Prior to the fertile phase cervical mucus is scant, thick, tacky, and breaks if stretched. The mucus becomes copious, clear, fluid, transparent, glossy and will stretch considerably between two fingers by the time of ovulation. After the fertile phase ends, mucus becomes scant, thick, opaque and non-stretchy again and the sensation of dryness will have returned. The fertile phase begins when any change towards a sensation of moisture or the quality of inspected mucus develops. It ends when three days of dryness or return to non-fertile mucus have been seen. Frequent inspection and charting are essential.

The cervical palpation method

This relies on the changes in cervical position and texture as well as the state of the cervical external os. After menstruation, the cervix lies low in the vagina, feels tough and the os is closed. As ovulation approaches the cervix rises higher into the pelvis, perhaps even out of reach, and the os opens. After the fertile phase is passed these changes regress. As with the cervical mucus method, frequent observation and charting is required. It is suggested that cervical examination can be performed by the woman's partner if the couple wish.

Lactational amenorrhoea method (LAM)

This can be practised for the first six months following childbirth in women who breast feed. It will considerably reduce their already reduced fertility. It is, however, valid only for the first six months and there are several requirements that must be met if the method is to be effective. The new-born baby should be put to the breast as soon after birth as possible and left with the mother for as long as possible. Feeding should be frequent, exclusively from the breast and practised on demand day and night. If the method is to continue after six months of age when supplements are introduced feeding should be given from the breast before the supplements are offered.

The 'double-check' method

This relies on a cocktail of techniques to predict the beginning and the end of the fertile phase. To predict the onset of the fertile phase choose from:

- calendar calculation (shortest cycle −19), checked previously with BBT charts
- first mucus symptom or sign
- cervical palpation

To predict the end of the fertile phase choose whichever is the later:

- sustained temperature shift of three days
- peak mucus plus four days

The symptothermal method

This method uses BBT charts plus cervical mucus or cervical changes or the calendar method.

There are other self-explanatory terms in use; calculothermal, mucothermal, Multiple Index Method.

The Persona

In 1996, Unipath launched a new contraceptive device, the Persona. The device is a very neatly packaged microcomputer incorporating a stick which the woman uses to test her urine. The device is set up to analyse the urine for luteinising hormone and oestrone-3-glucuronide, a metabolite of oestradiol. The device programme is initiated when the M button is pressed on the first day of the woman's period. A yellow light shows on the days the woman has to test her urine, green light shows on days when unprotected intercourse is safe and a red light when it is not. On these red days, abstinence or a barrier form of contraception should be employed.

At the time of writing, no published trials on the Persona have reached the public domain. However, the manufacturers and representatives of the British Medical Devices Agency (MDA) who have seen trial data concur that it has a 94% success rate per annum. That is, for every one hundred women using this method for contraception, six will become pregnant each year. This is equivalent to one in every seventeen users each year. This is a higher failure rate than with conscientious condom usage.

To quote the MDA 'While a useful addition to the range of contraceptive choices, Persona is basically a test-based form of the rhythm method of contraception. However, due to its technological basis, expectations of Persona may be higher than for other forms of contraception'.

The device is not NHS prescribable and costs around £50.00 to buy. Test sticks cost around a further £10.00 per month.

Points:

- **Persona is unsuitable for** women whose menstrual cycle length falls outside 23–35 days, breast feeders, users of oral contraceptives, infertility treatments and HRT. It is also unsuitable for women with liver or kidney complaints, women with polycystic ovary syndrome and women for whom pregnancy is contraindicated (eg. on chemotherapy)
- **Persona cannot be relied upon if** the woman uses certain medication: oestrogens, anti-oestrogens, progestins, progesterone, gonadotrophins, gonadotrophin releasing analogues, tetracycline (but not doxycycline or oxytetracycline) and the herbal medicine Vitex Agnus Castus
- **Emergency contraception** (EC): The Faculty of Family Planning of the Royal College of Obstetricians advise in their 'Recommendations for Clinical Practice: Emergency Contraception' (RCOG, 1998) that women using hormonal EC who also use the Persona should not use the device as a guide for contraception until two cycles lasting between 23–35 days have occurred subsequent to the cycle in which EC was used.
- **Contact/Helpline numbers**:
  - Technical questions helpline 0990 134430 (or: www.unipath.com/persona2)
  - Customer helpline 0345 447744
  - Unipath state in their literature that 'All Boots healthcare staff have been fully trained to answer questions about Persona'
- **References**:
  - Persona Professional Information Pack, 1997
  - Persona Contraceptive Device. Medicines Devices Agency, Jan 1998
  - Warning on contraceptive devices given, Mayor S (News), *Br Med J* 1998, **316**: 168
  - *Recommendations for Clinical Practice: Emergency Contraception* (FFP of RCOG, 1998)

Emergency contraception

See *Tables 3.9–3.11*. The therapeutic abortion rate in the UK testifies to the under-use of emergency contraception. All who deal with contraception, especially in younger women, should preach the message of emergency contraception. Several studies have shown that in addition to widespread ignorance among women of emergency contraception, health services place barriers to its delivery especially at weekends (the time of greatest need) when family planning clinics are shut and GPs may be reluctant to carry supplies or see women who have had unprotected coitus. Women attending A&E departments find doctors with no family planning experience and frequently a judgemental attitude. Organisation of the service, including education of receptionists and other ancillary staff, is recommended. We need to do better. The options are:

- **Oestrogen/progestogen EC**
- **Progestogen only EC**
- **IUD EC**

Table 3.9: Emergency contraception

Method	Timing	Contraindications*	Failure rate
Oestrogen/progestin 'Yuzpe method'	up to 72 hours after intercourse	severe focal migraine	3.2%
Progestin only	within 72 hours of intercourse	progestogen allergy	1.1%
IUD	up to 5 days after expected date of ovulation	usual IUD contraindications	<1%

* Most contraindications are relative for such short use. Severe focal migraine is an absolute contraindication for oestrogens

Oestrogen/progestogen emergency contraception (The Yuzpe method):

- **Treatment**: tabs ethinyloestradiol 50 mcg/ levonorgestrel 250 mcg x 2 stat with food. Repeat dose 12 hours later. Failure rates rise as the time between intercourse and the first dose lengthens. Recent evidence suggests it rises by 50% for every twelve hours delay
- **Formulations**: PC4 (Ovran is identical but comes with 21 tabs per pack and without a patient information leaflet on EC)
- **Indications**: for contraception after unprotected sexual intercourse. Can be used up to 72 hours after the episode. If previous episodes of unprotected intercourse have occurred in the same cycle more than 72 hours ago then this method is inappropriate
- **Cautions**: high dose oestrogens can cause vomiting. Take medication with food. Consider use of anti-emetic. If vomiting occurs within three hours of either dose it should be repeated or another method considered. Ectopic pregnancy is at the very least not prevented by the Yuzpe method. There is dispute whether it can cause ectopic pregnancy. In any case, it should be mentioned to the woman so that if menstruation is delayed or if abdominal pain develops she can seek urgent review. Coitus after previous use of EC in the same cycle will not be covered. A repeat prescription should be given if appropriate
- **Contraindications**: pregnancy, focal or crescendo migraine, thromboembolic disease. Longer term risks of high dose oestrogens, eg. coronary artery disease are not considered contraindications
- **Interactions**: enzyme inducing drugs. With these it is suggested that double the usual dose is given, ie. four tabs stat and repeat in twelve hours, or that another method is used
- **Follow up**: mandatory if abdominal pain develops. Strongly advised to ensure that pregnancy has not occurred despite EC precautions. Contraception in the longer term should be addressed.

Progestogen-only emergency contraception:

- **Treatment**: Previously known as the Ho and Kwan method; levonorgestrel, two stat doses of 750 mcg 12 hours apart with first dose within 72 hours of intercourse
- **Formulations**: see table
- **Indications**: for contraception after unprotected sexual intercourse. Can be used up to 72 hours after the episode. If previous episodes of unprotected intercourse have occurred in the same cycle more than 72 hours ago then this method is inappropriate
- **Cautions**: ensure that no other episodes of unprotected intercourse occurred in same cycle more than72 hours previously. Coitus after previous use of EC in the same cycle will not be covered. A repeat prescription should be given if appropriate
- **Contraindications**: pregnancy. Allergy to levonorgestrel

- **Interactions**: Enzyme inducing drugs; no data on how to circumvent this hazard
- **Follow up**: As for the Yuzpe method.

A World Health Organization trial of levonorgestrel only emergency contraception has found that it is better at preventing pregnancy and is less likely to cause nausea and vomiting than the Yuzpe regime using high dose combined pills. The Yuzpe regime of emergency contraception was found to have an overall pregnancy rate of 3.2%, compared with just 1.1% for the progestogen only levonorgestrel method. Success rates were better for both methods the sooner after intercourse they were taken, but the levonorgestrel method outperformed the Yuzpe regime in all time periods. Nausea and vomiting were significantly more common in women assigned to the Yuzpe regime. Levonorgestrel is currently only available in 30 and 37.5 mcg tablets. The regime requires two stat doses of 750 mcg twelve hours apart, that is either 25 or 20 depending on tablet strength, repeated 12 hours later (Guillebaud J, 1998; *Task Force on Postovulatory Methods of Fertility Regulation*, 1998). See *Tables 3.10–3.11.*

Table 3.10: Pregnancy rates for Yuzpe and POP/EC methods

Timing of 1st dose	Yuzpe regime	LNG method
<24 hours	1.96%	0.44%
24–48 hours	4.05%	1.18%
49–72 hours	4.67%	2.67%
Overall (0–72 hours)	3.2%	1.1%

Table 3.11: POP/EC; Practical prescribing advice

Product	Pack data	Emergency contraception regime
Microval	35 x levonorgestrel 30 mcg	25 tabs stat repeat after 12 hours
Norgestron	35 x levonorgestrel 30 mcg	25 tabs stat repeat after 12 hours
Neogest	35 x norgestrel 75 mcg (equivalent to levonorgestrel 37.5 mcg)	20 tabs stat repeat after 12 hours

Notes:
Prescribing point: Give the patient two packs of levonorgestrel 'mini-pills'. Advise the patient to take twenty-five tablets (or twenty in the case of Neogest) in one go. To avoid confusion discard the remaining tablets and repeat the dose twelve hours later with a new packet. This method remains unlicensed (outside Marketing Authorisation) and, as such, requires that the patients be aware of this, that the prescriber keeps a register of its prescription that can be audited at a later date and that the prescriber accepts full medico-legal responsibility (Recommendations for Clinical Practice: Emergency Contraception. FFP&RH of the RCOG. November 1998)
Stop press: A licensed two dose levonorgestrel EC pack is due to be launced in the UK early 2000. It is anticipated that Schering PC4 will be withdrawn thereafter

IUD emergency contraception

- **Treatment**: fitting of a copper IUD (Mirena not suitable)
- **Formulations**: any copper-containing IUD. For short term use choice will depend on ease of fitting especially in nulliparous women, and cost. For women considering longer term use one of the long life IUDs should be selected (see above in IUD section)

- **Indications**: unprotected intercourse. May be fitted up to five days after the expected date of ovulation. This date is calculated as nine days prior to the next expected period (day 21 in a 28-day cycle). Can be left *in situ* after the next period and used as principal mode of contraception (see section on IUD above)
- **Cautions**: vaginal examination vital to exclude pelvic tenderness and other contraindications of IUD
- **Contraindications**: pregnancy and all the other contraindications mentioned in the section on IUDs above. Pelvic infection and in circumstances where ectopic gestation is predisposed are particularly important, eg. following rape because of risk of STD
- **Interactions**: none for short term use
- **Follow up**: as for Yuzpe method

References

Connolly W (1994) *World Tour of Scotland*. BBC Presentations, London

Dyer C (1985) Contraceptives and the under 16s: House of Lords ruling. *Br Med J* **291**: 1208–9

Grodstein F *et al* (1994) A prospective study of symptomatic gallstones in women: relation with oral contraceptives and other risk factors. *Obstet Gynecol* **84**: 207–14

Guillebaud J (1994) *Contraception: Your Questions Answered*, 2nd edn (revised). Churchill Livingstone, London

Guillebaud J (1998) Time for emergency contraception with levonorgestrel alone (commentary). *Lancet* **352**: 416

Korver T, Goorissen E, Guillebaud J (1995) The combined oral contraceptive pill: what advice should we give when tablets are missed? *Br J Obstet Gynaecol* **102**: 601–7

Lewis MA *et al* (1996) Third generation oral contraceptives and the risk of myocardial infarction: an international case-control study. *Br Med J* **312**: 88–90

Rauman-Wilms L *et al* (1995) Female genital effects of first trimester sex hormone exposure: a meta-analysis. *Obstet Gynecol* **85**: 141–9

Rookus MA, van Leeuwen FE (1994) Oral contraception and the risk of breast cancer in women aged 20–54 years. *Lancet* **344**: 844–51

Schering Health Care Ltd (1995) Company communication to GPs

Scientific Committee of The Faculty of Family Planning and Reproductive Health Care (1996) Guidelines for prescribing combined oral contraceptives. *Br Med J* **312**: 121

Spitzer WO *et al* (1996) Third generation oral contraceptives and the risk of venous thromboembolic disorders: an international case-control study. *Br Med J* **312**: 83–8

Szarewski A, Guillebaud J (1994) *Contraception: a user's handbook*.Oxford University Press, Oxford

Tacchi D (on behalf of the National Association of Family Planning Doctors) (1990) IUD fitting in the over 40-year-olds, (letter). *Lancet* **336**: 182

Task Force on Postovulatory Methods of Fertility Regulation (1998) Randomised trial of levonorgestrel versus the Yuzpe regime of combined oral contraceptives for emergency contraception. *Lancet* **352**: 428–433

Recommended reading

Guillebaud J (1994) *Contraception: Your Questions Answered*, 2 edn (revised). Churchill Livingstone, London

Szarewski A, Guillebaud J (1994) *Contraception: A User's Handbook*. Oxford University Press, Oxford

Loudon N, Glasier A, Gebbie A (eds) (1995) *Handbook of Family Planning and Reproductive Health Care*, 3 edn. Churchill Livingstone, London

Carter Y, Moss C, Weyman A (eds) (1998) *RCGP Handbook of Sexual Health in Primary Care*. RCGP, London

4
preconceptual care

Many women resolve to improve their health when they become pregnant. But by the time some have found out they have conceived, organogenesis has occurred and the full potential of another human being may already have been compromised. Preconceptual care, like emergency contraception, should not just be available; it must be prospectively offered. Well woman check-up, attendance for contraception and even postnatal visits and child immunisation clinics provide excellent opportunities for advertising preconceptual wares when women may be most receptive. Data is presented alphabetically under three headings.

Chapter contents

aims   *check-lists*
clinical questions   *references and further reading*

Aims

- **alcohol reduction or elimination**: it is prudent to advise abstinence during the first trimester and modest intake thereafter (1–2 units per day maximum)

- **caffeine**: there is evidence that fecundity is reduced in women with a heavy intake of caffeine (eight cups of coffee per day, or equivalent). Spontaneous abortion may also be more common in women who take a large amount of caffeine each day

- **collection of baseline data** which can be used for comparative purposes during and after the hoped for pregnancy (eg. Rubella antibody status, iron status, blood group)

- **depressive disorder** and psychiatric conditions should be sensitively discussed. Mood changes are well known developments in the puerperium but can also occur during pregnancy. Cessation of psychotropic drugs carries a high risk of relapse in women with depressive disorder and continuation or even initiation of therapy during pregnancy is often advisable (see *Chapter 6*, section on puerperal affective disorders)

- **diabetes mellitus** is discussed below. Poor control carries a massive increase in the risk of fetal abnormality. Preconceptual workup in a combined clinic (obstetric and diabetologist) is strongly recommended

- **epilepsy** is discussed below and in *Chapter 7*. Many of the drugs used in controlling epileptic seizures are teratogenic. Preconceptual counselling is strongly recommended by the CSM. The preconceptual involvement of an obstetrician with an interest and the neurologist is strongly recommended. Preconceptual folic acid supplementation is vital. The recommended pre-conceptual dose is a full 5 mg/day. Early pregnancy screening for NTD is advisable. See *Chapter 7* for drug lists

- **general worries** can be addressed and explored and previous obstetric problems may be particularly relevant

- **nutritional advice** can be given. There are helpful leaflets (see further reading) that can be used to supplement any verbal advice although folate rich foods are no substitute for folic acid tablets

- **optimise health** sounds grand but includes attention to current or potential illnesses and medications, eg. asthma or thyroid disease. Problems may be spotted on examination that can be attended to, so improving the chance of a happy outcome in future pregnancies, eg. hypertension or anaemia

- **screening:** when future pregnancy is being discussed there is an excellent opportunity to promote screening. The principal screen is of course cervical cytology. In certain circumstances other conditions may need screening for, eg. sickle cell trait, thalassaemia or genetic disorder

- **smoking advice:** smoking is harmful in pregnancy. There is evidence that placentation is effected before the first missed period, indicating that smoking cessation when pregnancy is confirmed is too late. Indeed the follicular fluid that bathes the oocyte before ovulation is contaminated by cotinine, a metabolite of nicotine in smokers

---

Clinical questions

- **alcohol** is a weak teratogen in small doses. Regular heavy drinking is the cause of the fetal alcohol syndrome. Ideally, alcohol should not be taken when trying to conceive and drinking during pregnancy, especially the first trimester, is inadvisable

- **bacterial vaginosis** is associated with mid-trimester abortion and preterm labour. Symptomatic women should be treated. The case for screening preconceptually remains open. Trials in asymptomatic pregnant women have shown benefit. If asymptomatic BV is found incidentally before pregnancy it would be difficult to defend not eradicating it before conception

- **cats** see toxoplasmosis

- **cytomegalovirus** (CMV): this is discussed in *Chapter 6*. There is no routine indication for checking it before pregnancy

- **diabetes mellitus** is discussed more fully in *Chapter 7*. Briefly, it is proven that poorly controlled diabetes is associated with a massive increase in risk of fetal abnormality. Rigorous euglycaemic control for several months before conception can reduce the fetal abnormality rate to one that is equivalent to the general population

- **folic acid supplementation** has been shown to reduce the incidence of neural tube defect affected pregnancies (Medical Research Council, 1991). The current advice is that all women should be advised to take a small supplement of folic acid (400 mcg/day) from the time that they decide to try to become pregnant until the twelfth week of pregnancy (Department of Health, 1992). Folic acid tablets are recommended as folate rich foods may not effectively increase red-cell folate levels (Cuskelly *et al*, 1996). Supplementation is especially important in women taking anti-convulsant medication who should also take a higher dose (5 mg/day). Women who conceive without folic acid supplementation should start taking it as soon as possible and continue until twelve weeks gestation. The neural tube however closes at six weeks. For a good brief review see Trewinnard (1996)

- **gardening** see toxoplasmosis and listeriosis

- **genetic questions** can be usefully addressed preconceptually. Many women will be interested to hear about the place of antenatal diagnostic testing for chromosome anomaly. Some women will have relevant factors in their personal, ethnic or family history. Most commonly there may be a family history of cystic fibrosis or Down's syndrome. It is usual to arrange counselling in such instances with a gynaecologist with a special interest, or a geneticist. Many obstetric units now run combined clinics with multi-disciplinary input

- **healthy eating** involves ensuring an adequate intake of essential nutrients and the avoidance of teratogens and food-borne infections. There are useful advisory leaflets that can be given to women planning pregnancy (see further reading below). During pregnancy it is important to avoid an excessive intake of Vitamin A. Listeriosis and toxoplasmosis are uncommon but serious food-borne pathogens

- **listeriosis** can cause serious fetal infection which can result in intrauterine death or handicap. Listeria monocytogenes is a Gram (+) rod, a gut commencal in 20% of the population and present in soil and on soiled vegetables. It is also found occasionally in paté, soft cheeses and in prepared salads. It can proliferate at temperatures as low as 6°C (see listeriosis, *Chapter 6*)

- **past obstetric problems** should always be inquired about. This includes prior history of miscarriage and termination of pregnancy. If areas of difficulty or distress are highlighted then consultation with an obstetrician, midwife or even a paediatrician can be arranged. Previous uncomplicated vaginal termination of pregnancy is not considered a physical risk factor for future pregnancy

- **rubella status** must be checked before pregnancy. A history of prior vaccination does not mean that protection is absolute. A previous history of German measles is a poor predictor of rubella antibody status. There have been reports of antibody levels dropping over time and so it is probably advisable to check rubella antibody status before each pregnancy. Rubella vaccine is contraindicated in pregnancy which should be avoided for three months after the injection of the live vaccine. Inadvertent vaccination during or just before pregnancy has not however been shown to be teratogenic

- **sheep** can be vectors for listeriosis, toxoplasmosis as well as *chlamydia psiticci*, a cause of abortion in both lambs and humans. Women contemplating pregnancy, especially those from rural areas and the farming community, should be alert to these hazards. Febrile illness, which can occur at any stage in pregnancy, should prompt referral for investigation in susceptible individuals

- **tobacco** in the form of cigarettes is toxic in pregnancy. Placentation is compromised before the mother is aware of becoming pregnant. Indeed, cotinine can be isolated from ovarian follicles bathing the oocyte before ovulation. Fetal growth is compromised leading to small for dates babies. Smoking cessation should be advised and facilitated before conception. In those who cannot stop, smoking reduction without laying a burden of guilt upon the prospective mother is the aim

- *toxoplasma gondii* is a protozoa that is most commonly spread via cats' faeces. All soil, including dirty vegetables, should be considered contaminated. Women should wear gloves when gardening or handling soiled vegetables before and during pregnancy. Vegetables should be thoroughly washed before preparation. Similarly, hand washing after handling cats and other domestic animals is advisable. The disposal of cat litter should be delegated to others by women before and during pregnancy. The other principal source of toxoplasma infection is undercooked infected meat. Primary infection carries the risk of significant fetal infection which can result in congenital damage or even death Primary infection contracted just before pregnancy can cause transplacental infection. Congenital toxoplasmosis is however a rarity, affecting just 1:50,000 births in England and Wales in 1989/90

  Should women be screened for toxoplasma antibodies preconceptually? Certainly the detection of antibodies will be of some reassurance and the absence of antibodies will encourage risk avoidance strategies. The problem arises if seroconversion occurs during pregnancy. In France, where toxoplasmosis is more prevalent, antibody negative women have levels checked regularly throughout pregnancy. Seroconversion will be followed by the offer of further investigations which may include cordocentesis. As 50% of pregnancies will be unaffected by primary maternal infection, and as the drug treatments are used empirically, there is a significant dilemma surrounding the use of invasive tests which are attended by measurable morbidity and mortality. As it is, sero-surveillance for toxoplasmosis is not routinely offered through pregnancy in this country. While every affected child represents a tragedy, iatrogenic intrauterine death is a disaster. See 'General principles' in *Screening in gynaecology*', Chapter 1

- **Vitamin A** in high doses is teratogenic. It can cause facial clefting anomalies. Vitamin A is found in several vitamin supplements some of which may not carry a warning against their use in pregnancy. Vitamin A is also found at significant levels in liver and liver products. Advice against consumption of these products was given some years ago because of this. Some authorities however suggest that a ban is too harsh as less affluent women may obtain a good amount of nutrition from liver which is a cheap cut of meat. The current advice is that no more than one portion of liver or two portions of a liver product (eg. liver sausage) should be taken in any one week. The retinol group of drugs have similar restriction on their use before and during pregnancy (tretinoin, isotretinoin). See section on drug use before and during pregnancy, *Chapter 7*. β-carotene is not associated with anomaly

---

Check-lists

The problem with check-lists is that they can be a refuge of the thoughtless and a stick for the righteous to beat you with. The following are therefore neither protocols (suggesting omission is neglect) nor guidelines (suggesting protocols, but with less authority). They are check-lists for you to consider and adapt for each individual who presents.

Preconceptual checklists — history

- **ethnicity** must be considered if relevant. Thalassaemia in couples of Mediterranean and Asian origin may be important. Certain groups, for example Askenazi Jews, have particularly high rates of congenital disorder and others, for example of Pakistani origin, may be married to close relatives increasing the manifestation of recessive traits

- **family history** can be critical where congenital disorder is concerned. In some cases insight into family circumstances may prompt the offer of specialist help from health visitors, midwives and social workers

- **medication** must be considered. Do not forget the extensive range of over-the-counter preparations. Common individual drugs and conditions that are seen in women in their childbearing years are discussed in *Chapter 7*. The *BNF* has listings on the effects of drugs in pregnancy. If doubt remains the *Data Sheet Compendium* or your local drug information service should be consulted. Responsibility rests with the prescriber

- **menstrual history** may indicate a possible impediment to fertility. It is also useful data in calculating gestational age in early pregnancy before confirmatory scanning

- **obstetric history** should always be elucidated. Some problems are recurrent in nature, others are related to high parity

- **occupational history** is important. Some occupations carry pregnancy risks, eg. CMV sero-negative nursery nurses, those handling toxic chemicals or drugs, veterinarians and farm workers involved in handling sheep

- **past medical history,** especially of epilepsy, diabetes, cardiac, hepatic and renal disorder. A complete list of relevant conditions would be unwieldy. Most women will be healthy and PMH will not be applicable

- **sexually transmitted disease** history should be tactfully touched upon. Particular infections are discussed in *Chapters 6* and *7*. Of particular importance are gonococcal and herpes virus infections, *condylomata accuminata* and, of course, HIV. Bacterial vaginosis, although not a classical STD, is also of relevance (see above)

Preconceptual check-lists — examination

- **abdominal examination** may reveal organomegaly, uterine fibroids, scars etc. An over-modest reaction may belie psychosexual problems

- **blood pressure** is possibly the most important single test for spotting a future pregnancy risk that is amenable to intervention. A vital baseline measure

- **breast examination** will not be indicated routinely. A breast examination is wise if a check has not been performed in the preceding two years

- **other systems** can be examined. There are suggestions that the spine should be checked so that physiotherapy can be obtained early if necessary; that the teeth are inspected as gum disease can progress rapidly and free dental care is available in pregnancy, and that the thyroid be palpated. Examination of the cardiovascular and respiratory systems are only indicated for those with appropriate symptoms or signs. The lack of hours in the day imposes limits

- **pelvic examination** will not be indicated routinely. Relevant symptoms or abdominal signs may prompt speculum and bimanual examination

- **weight/height/BMI** baseline measurements. Height is not a good predictor of obstetric performance 'the fetal head is the best pelvimeter'

Preconceptual check-lists — tests

- **CMV and toxoplasma antibodies** are contentious. Those in high risk categories (eg. nursery nurses and those with above average contact with infants and toddlers for CMV; veterinarians, livestock workers, farmers, those handling raw meat etc. for toxoplasmosis) may wish to know their antibody status. Finding antibodies is reassuring, their absence poses a dilemma. If in doubt consult an infectious diseases specialist

- **haemoglobin** and other tests for iron status become difficult to interpret in pregnancy. A blood count for baseline purposes and to identify those requiring pre-pregnancy iron supplementation (especially in those with menorrhagia, IUD contraception or numerous previous pregnancies) is advisable

- **HVS** should be taken if indicated clinically. In asymptomatic women there is, as yet, no proof that eradication of asymptomatic bacterial vaginosis is of benefit even though BV is implicated in late miscarriage and preterm labour. If a contemporaneous cervical smear result is not available, a smear test should be performed

- **MSU:** Asymptomatic bacteriuria can lead silently to pyelonephritis and renal scarring. Screening it out is reassuring. Testing for glycosuria and proteinuria is so simple it would be wrong to omit it

- **rhesus factor**: knowledge of Rhesus D status can be extremely helpful in the event of bleeding in pregnancy; 90% will be Rh-D positive

- **rubella antibody levels** should be known for all women contemplating pregnancy. It is prudent to have a rubella Ab check prior to each pregnancy as there are suggestions that immunity can wane

- **varicella** (chickenpox) can cause serious fetal, neonatal and maternal morbidity and even mortality (see Varicella-Zoster, *Chapter 6*). As yet, there is no national policy for immunising women pre-conceptually as is done for Rubella rather than waiting until disease develops and instituting passive immunisation with VZIG. The question is under review and it could become a baseline screening test in the future as it is now, for example, in the United States

Preconceptual check-lists — advice

- **avoidance of pathogenic micro-organisms** namely: toxoplasma, CMV, rubella, listeria and the organisms causing sexually transmitted disease. Primary maternal chickenpox, especially near or at term poses a severe risk to the fetus/neonate as well as to the mother

- **drugs and medication** must be reviewed. Further details can be found in *Chapters 6 and 7* on management of common medical conditions in pregnancy and in the section on illicit drug use in pregnancy

- **folic acid supplements** should be taken by all women trying to conceive and by all women who become pregnant, up to the twelfth week of pregnancy. It is suggested that advising women about folic acid supplementation should begin during school years. The dose is 400 mcg per day (5 mg/day for women taking anti-epileptic medication). Foods rich in folic acid should also be recommended, although there is evidence that naturally folate-rich foods do not adequately supplement for pre-conceptual purposes. There are excellent government produced leaflets for distribution

- **genetic tests** should be offered by geneticists. Exceptions might be the exclusion of certain traits, eg. thalassaemia or sickle cell

- **healthy eating** is summarised in government produced leaflets which should be available for distribution. Folate-rich foods, however, are no substitute for folic acid supplemetation tablets. Moderation in caffeine intake is advisable

- **tobacco and alcohol** should be minimised or, ideally, stopped before pregnancy. Reduction is better than no action. Reduction during the first trimester is especially advantageous

References and further reading

Cuskelly GJ, McNulty H, Scott JM (1996) Effect of increasing dietary folate on red-cell folate: implications for prevention of neural tube defects. *Lancet* **347**: 657–9

Department of Health (1991) *While You Are Pregnant. Safe Eating and How to Avoid Infection from Food and Animals*. HMSO, London

Department of Health (1992) *Folic Acid in the Prevention of Neural Tube Defects*. Report from an advisory group. HMSO, London

Health Education Authority (1996) *Folic Acid — What All Women Should Know* (there are leaflets for patients and a booklet 'A summary guide for health professionals'). HEA, London

Management and Prevention of Listeriosis and Food-borne Infection in Pregnancy. PL/CMO (92) 19

MRC Vitamin Study Research Group (1991) Prevention of neural tube defects: results of the Medical Research Council Vitamin Study. *Lancet* **338**: 131–7

Trewinnard K (1996) Periconceptual folic acid supplementation and the prevention of neural tube defects. *Br J Fam Planning* **22**: 36–7

5
infertility

It is estimated that one in ten couples are infertile and that one in six will have fertility difficulties at some stage in their lives. The distress that frustrated parenthood brings is immense. At one end it can be intensely rewarding to help a couple achieve their dreams and, at the other, counselling couples to come to terms with permanent childlessness is one of the most difficult areas for health professionals.

Chapter contents

definitions and causes

infertility workup in primary care

anti-oestrogen ovulation induction therapy

assisted conception

adoption

useful addresses

references and further reading

Definitions and causes

- **amenorrhoea**: the absence of menstruation for six or more months. Common causes include menopause which can occur prematurely, pregnancy, the polycystic ovary syndrome (PCOS) and hyperprolactinaemia

- **BBT**: Basal body temperature rises after ovulation, progesterone is thermogenic. A sustained rise implies ovulation may have occurred. There is argument on the usefulness of BBTs. It is certainly true that some couples find charting and the implied requirement to have intercourse emotionally wearing. A rise of 0.5°C sustained for at least 7 days is a positive result. A narrow range 'fertility thermometer' is required to measure this small shift in temperature which has to be recorded immediately on waking, before rising (or anything else, eg. cup of tea, sexual intercourse) each morning. Pyrexia, shift work, late rising at the weekend and alcohol the night before are all sources of error

- **cumulative conception rates:** In counselling couples on fertility matters the use of cumulative conception graphs can be very illuminating. The encounter between spermatozoon and oocyte is a random affair. While one can say that the chance of conception per cycle in couples with no impediment is 1:4, the same chance for success will attend each consecutive month of trying. Those who conceive in the first month are lucky; those who take twelve months are unlucky. And, so-called infertility may simply be a reflection of impatience with our low fecundity

- **fecundity**: the ability to conceive in any one cycle. It drops slowly after the age of 30
- **fertility**: the ability to conceive over a period of time. This also drops with age, but less rapidly than fecundity
- **FSH** (follicle stimulating hormone): the pituitary gonadotrophin that stimulates the follicle to ripen and the ovary to produce oestrogen. FSH is best measured in the first few days of the cycle. A very low FSH can imply hypothalamic suppression. FSH is a male gonado-trophin too. Sperm generation by Sertoli cells is under the control of FSH
- **follicular phase** begins after the onset of menstruation and ends at ovulation
- **infertility** is generally assumed to be a possibility after twelve months of regular intercourse without successful con-ception. In the presence of particular symptoms and signs (eg. menstrual disturbance or varicocele) investigation may be instituted much earlier. Sub-fertility is thought by some to be a more accurate term as infertility implies a retrospective absolute diagnosis. See cumulative conception rates, above
- **LH** (lutinizing hormone): a pituitary gonadotrophin secreted in a short pulse at the end of the follicular phase causing follicular rupture and ovum release; ovulation. Continual, rather than pulsatile, LH secretion will inhibit ovulation and may lead to metropathia haemorrhagica (see menstrual disturb-ance, *Chapter 1*). This is one of the major features of PCOS. In the male, LH is the Leidig cell gonadotrophin and it is concerned with testosterone production
- **luteal phase** begins at ovulation and ends when menstruation or pregnancy super-

venes. It is characterised by the production of progesterone from the ruptured ovulatory follicle (corpus luteum). No ovulation; no progesterone. Progesterone peaks a week after ovulation, a week before menstruation. Correctly timed progesterone assays over 30 nmol/l imply ovulation. A short luteal phase, or sub-optimal progesterone levels, imply luteal phase deficiency

- **menstrual cycle nomenclature** is vital for clear communication. Day 1 of the cycle is the first day of menstruation. Everything hinges on this. Ovulation occurs around fourteen days before menstruation, and peak progesterone levels occur around seven days before menstruation. Follicular phase length is variable and ovulation is a moveable feast
- **oligomenorrhoea** defines infrequent menstruation; occurring between 6–26 weeks
- **ovulation induction** at the primary care level involves the use of anti-oestrogens (eg. clomiphene). At the secondary/ tertiary level pituitary down-regulation with hypothalamic hormonal analogues and gonadotrophin injections are available at considerable expense both fiscal and emotional
- **progesterone challenge test** is occasionally indicated to test the oestrogenic status of amenorrhoeic women. The test involves taking medroxyprogesterone acetate 5 mg/day for five days. A menstrual response in the following week implies good oestro-genisation and augurs well for clomiphene therapy. It can also be used to assess endometrial function in cases where Asherman's syndrome is suspected (loss of endometrium due to infection, ablation or curettage; may be associated with intrauterine adhesions)

- **social history** relates to the suitability of the couple to be parents. Inevitably, a degree of subjective judgement is involved, although there will be circumstances where a health professional may not wish to be involved in assisting those unsuited to parenthood with their infertility (eg. convicted paedophiles or perhaps couples with children already in care). If in doubt consult a fertility specialist for advice and perhaps suggest counselling of the couple concerned

Common causes of infertility

- **ovulation failure** may be suspected in the presence of menstrual disturbance, especially oligoamenorrhoea. Anovulation is physiological at the menopause and during lactation. Pathological causes include polycystic ovary syndrome (PCOS), weight-related hypothalamic causes (anorexia nervosa, athletes) and hyperprolactinaemia. Apart from menopausal ovulation failure, which may be premature, ovulatory failure is frequently amenable to therapy. Ovulation failure accounted for 21% of all cases of infertility in a study by Hull (1992)

- **obstruction** of the fallopian tubes accounted for around 14% in Hull's study. Tubal surgery and IVF/ET are the treatment options although a significant number of women conceive after hysterosalpingography. A history of pelvic infection (eg. peritonitis or chlamydial infection) is suggestive. In an asymptomatic woman with regular periods and whose partner has a good seminal fluid result it is the most likely of the differential diagnoses. Male obstructive problems are less common. They cause azoospermia in the presence of a normal FSH level

- **sperm problems** are the largest single identifiable cause of infertility (24% in Hull's study) and require a sophisticated workup (tertiary level care). The traditional 'sperm count' is poorly predictive of male fertility. The sperm production cycle is around ten weeks long. If a poor sperm count result is obtained, wait two months or more before repeating. Sperm problems can be caused by drugs including tobacco, alcohol and β-blockers which impede the propulsion system, scrotal varicocele and other conditions that elevate testicular temperature, as well as previous infection (especially mumps). A past history of inguinal hernia repair or orchidopexy can be important. Sertoli (sperm producing) cell failure will cause oligoazoospermia and is associated with a high FSH level

- **endometriosis** accounted for 6% of cases in Hull's study and is characterised by pelvic pain, dysmenorrhoea, dyspareunia and infertility. Ectopic endometrium, even in small amounts, seems 'toxic' to the fertility process. Endometriosis can cause tubal damage too, although IVF/ET is not compromised. Endometriotic deposits can be removed at the time of diagnostic laparoscopy

- **mucus defects** (cervical mucus) can cause infertility either because its character is not conducive to sperm sustenance and transport or because anti-sperm antibodies are present. Curiously anti-sperm antibodies can be present in the semen too (secondary/tertiary care problem). Intra-uterine or intra-tubal insemination (IUI and ITI) can overcome this problem

- **unexplained infertility** frustratingly accounted for 28% of all cases in Hull's study. IVF/ET is being seen increasingly as a test as well as a treatment for this condition. Empirical treatment with clomiphene is advocated by some gynaecologists as is IUI/ITI

- **small print** and other causes of infertility are legion. They include coital failure which was suspected in around 6% of cases in Hull's study; the postcoital test is sensitive in detecting this.

Genital tract anomaly, autoimmune disease and resistant ovary syndrome are a few of the many causes of infertility. In some women, the use of NSAIDs can interfere with ovulation and produce the luteinized unruptured follicle (LUF) syndrome. Cessation of therapy or at least avoiding use of NSAIDs around ovulation time can avert this problem

Infertility workup in primary care

This section is intended to provide check-lists, not protocols or rigid guidelines. Although some tests will be universally applicable, most should be reserved for use where justifiably indicated.

Female infertility workup checklist

Choose tests that will provide answers to prospective questions. Some tests eg. HIV may be required prior to entry to a tertiary care programme, especially if gamete donation is involved.

- full medical and obstetric history
- social history
- drug history
- menstrual/coital diary
- blood pressure
- BMI (kg/m^2)
- abdominal examination
- pelvic examination
- vaginal/cervix swabs including chlamydia
- cervical cytology
- MSU

- FBC
- FSH (early follicular phase)
- LH (early follicular phase)
- progesterone (mid-luteal phase)
- oestradiol
- prolactin (stress hormone, repeat if raised)
- TSH
- karyotype, eg. if Turner's suspected
- rubella antibody status
- HIV/Hep B status for some IVF units
- syphilis and chlamydia serology

Male infertility workup checklist

- full medical and paternity history
- social history
- occupational history
- drug history
- blood pressure
- BMI (kg/m^2)
- abdominal examination
- genital examination
- testicular volume is estimated using graded wooden ovoids

- rectal/prostate examination
- MSU
- sperm count is most helpful if azoospermia is found, otherwise a poor predictor of fertility
- detailed seminal analysis
- FSH and LH
- testosterone
- karyotype, eg. suspected Klienfelters
- HIV/Hep B status (may be required in some units)

Male infertility workup check-list

The interview and examination of male partners is generally less well attended to than it should be in primary care . The couple, and not just the woman, is sub-fertile. In some cases there will be impediments in both parties. It does in fact 'take two' (Gaye and Weston, 1967).

WHO values for seminal analysis (1992)

volume	≥2ml
pH	7.2–8.0
concentration	≥20 million sperm/ml
total count	≥40 million
motility	≥50% showing forward progression
morphology	≥30% normal forms
vitality	≥75% live sperms
white cell count	<1 million/ml

Anti-oestrogen ovulation induction therapy

This is the one fertility treatment that primary care doctors can prescribe and supervise themselves. It is indicated in well oestrogenised anovulatory women. In fact, some gynaecologists use it empirically in women who have cycles that are irregular or slightly longer than average and in unexplained infertility. The action of the anti-oestrogen is on the pituitary. It promotes appropriate gonadotrophin secretion and 62% of well oestrogenised women will ovulate in the first cycle (86% after three cycles).

- **preparations**: clomiphene, tamoxifen and cyclofenil. Only clomiphene is used widely for infertility in primary care

- **prerequisites**: an intact hypothalamic-pituitary-ovarian axis. Poor results in hypo-oestrogenised states. Precede with preconceptual care and ensure rubella antibodies are present and folic acid is being given

- **dose**: clomiphene 25–150 mg/day. Responses are inconsistent

- **regime**: commence with 50 mg/day for five days beginning on day 2 of the cycle. If satisfactory ovulatory response results, continue for up to six cycles. If sub-optimal response, increase dose to 75 mg, 100 mg or 150 mg (maximum) per day for the five days

- **monitoring** a good luteal response with mid-luteal progesterone >40 nmol/l. This is higher than the unstimulated threshold. Periodical pelvic examination to exclude the development of ovarian cysts (ovarian hyperstimulation)

- **duration of therapy** is generally for up to six months. Clomiphene therapy can be instituted and continued while awaiting a specialist opinion. If ovulation is not stimulated, or if conception fails to occur, specialist assistance will be required

- **multiple gestation risk**: unlike gonadotrophin therapy, anti-oestrogens are associated with a low risk of multiple pregnancy, hence their safety in primary care. The twin pregnancy rate is only slightly higher than in spontaneous pregnancies

- **ovarian hyperstimulation risk**: unlike gonadotrophin therapy, anti-oestrogens are associated with a very low risk of ovarian hyperstimulation, hence their safety in primary care. Hyperstimulation causes ovarian cyst development and ascites. The development of abdominal symptoms or the formation of ovarian cysts requires prompt attention and if hyperstimulation is suspected, seek specialist involvement

- **ovarian cancer**: there are suggestions that incessant ovulation/superovulation increases the risk of ovarian cancer. It is certainly true that ovulation suppression with, for example, the combined oral contraceptive pill reduces the incidence of ovarian cancer. It would therefore be prudent for primary care professionals to restrict their use of clomiphene to six cycles

---

Assisted conception

This is a tertiary care service. Although primary care professionals will not be expected to prescribe or manage cases an awareness of the services is helpful. A few treatments may be administered in primary care. Listed below are a few of the more commonly used terms. New ones are constantly appearing as the technology advances/develops.

- **Donor insemination** is self-descriptive. Donors are anonymous, selected phenotypically and screened for potential genetic and infectious hazards (including HIV and Hep B)

- **Down-regulation** involves suppressing the pituitary with hypothalamic analogues (GnRH) so that natural cyclical activity stops. The use of exogenous gonadotrophins is thus simplified

- **Embryo** describes fertilised oocytes that have undergone a few cell divisions. These are at the pre-implantation stage

- **ET:** embryo transfer describes the placing of a fertilised oocyte into the fallopian tube or uterus

- **GnRH:** gonadotrophin releasing hormone or LHRH (luteinizing hormone releasing hormone) is secreted by the hypothalamus. The synthetic analogues initially stimulate the pituitary gonadotrophs before suppressing them. GnRH and its synthetic analogues suppress the pituitary and consequently the ovary (and testis). They are used in the treatment of endometriosis and prostatic cancer as well as infertility. The

available GnRH analogues are buserelin, goserelin, leuprorelin acetate and nafarelin. They are given as injections or as nasal sprays. They are a secondary/tertiary care treatment

- **GIFT:** gamete intra-fallopian transfer; one of the catchiest acronyms ever devised. Basically, sperm is introduced into the fallopian tube through the fimbrial opening at laparoscopy

- **ICSI:** intracytoplasmic sperm injection; a method of insemination where a single sperm is helped to unite with the oocyte by microdissection of the cumulus and zona pellucida and injected into the cytoplasm of the oocyte. There is increasing evidence that the congenital abnormality rate is higher in ICSI babies than in the general population

- **ITI:** intra-tubal insemination. This treatment is being used increasingly in unexplained infertility and where there is a male factor

- **IUI:** intra-uterine insemination. This treatment is being used in unexplained infertility and where there is a male factor

- **IVF**: *in-vitro* fertilisation; the test tube bit of the 'test tube baby'
- **Luteal support** may be used following ovulation induction, ET or other fertility treatments including in some cases the use of clomiphene. It involves the use of progesterone (Cyclogest pessaries, Crinone gel or, more commonly, Gestone injection) or chorionic gonadotrophin (hCG) injections. A secondary/tertiary care treatment, but may be administered in primary care by arrangement
- **Ovum donation** is an option for women who have undergone a premature menopause, had oophorectomy or for genetic reasons. Analogous to donor insemination. The oocyte can be transferred to the fallopian tube mimicking ovulation or, more commonly, fertilised *in-vitro* prior to embryo transfer
- **Pregnancy reduction** involves the killing of one or more fetuses, usually by intracardiac injection and late in the first trimester. The procedure may be an option in high-grade multiple pregnancy where there is great risk of miscarriage or very premature labour and the loss of the entire pregnancy. Reduction of say sextuplets to twins will increase the take home baby rate as well as reduce the incidence of prematurity induced damage to survivors. Reduction of normal twin pregnancies to singletons is a different social and moral question
- **Surrogacy** involves one woman gestating for another. Various combinations of gametes are possible. The oocyte may be the infertile woman's, from a donor or from the surrogate mother. The sperm can be the infertile couple's or from a donor. Insemination can take place *in-vitro*, by artificial IUI or (in an unregulated arrangement) by natural sexual intercourse. A tertiary care procedure when regulated
- **ZIFT**: zygote intra-fallopian transfer. Like GIFT but an embryo is transferred rather than sperm

Adoption

A very special area of human endeavour. In the seriously sub-fertile it is a valuable option. The remit of the adopting agencies is to find suitable families for children and not to find suitable children for the childless, ie. it is very definitely child-centred. It should be on the agenda in managing all cases of infertility although only in a few cases will it be a preferred choice or viable option. See useful addresses below.

Useful addresses

- ISSUE (the national fertility association) Independent Infertility Support and Self-Help
  Unit 9, 509 Aldridge Road, Great Barr Birmingham, B44 8NA
- CHILD (self-help advice for couples)
  Room 219, Caledonian House
  98 The Centre, Feltham
  Middlesex, TW13 4BH
- The Family Planning Association
  27 Mortimer Street
  London N1N 7RJ
- British Agencies for Adoption and Fostering (BAAF)
  11 Southwark Street
  London SE1 1RQ

References and further reading

Gaye M, Weston K (1967) It Takes Two. In: Gambaccini P, Rice T, eds. *British Book of Hit Singles, 8 edn.* Guinness Publishing, Middlesex

Hull MGR (1992) *Infertility Treatments: Needs and Effectiveness.* A Report from the University of Bristol, Department of Obstetrics and Gynaecology, Bristol

Hull MGR *et al* (1986) Population study of causes, treatment and outcome of infertility. *Br Med J* **291**: 1693

pregnancy and the puerperium (1) consequential conditions

Pregnancy is a physiological condition and delivery a natural event. Sadly, physiology and nature are not always kind and can slide, sometimes barely perceptibly, sometimes with frightening rapidity, into pathology and morbidity. Care in pregnancy and the puerperium is complicated by accumulated unenlightening anecdotage and socio-political warfare among both healthcare professionals and interested members of the public. The management of labour and delivery is not considered a basic primary care topic (although many primary care professionals will be involved in delivering this secondary care service) and is beyond the scope of this chapter.

Data for the primary care professional on the common or important antenatal problem areas are listed alphabetically. The 'Big Five' antenatal complications are altered glucose tolerance, anaemia, antepartum haemorrhage, pregnancy induced hypertension and urinary tract infection.

Chapter contents

Tables

Altered glucose tolerance

Altered glucose tolerance is one of the big five antenatal disorders. One has to distinguish between the diabetic woman who plans to become pregnant, the diabetic woman who is pregnant and the woman who becomes or behaves as a diabetic after she becomes pregnant. There is a link between gestational diabetes mellitus (GDM) and the risk of developing non-gestational diabetes in the future.

Terminology

- **euglycaemia**: the condition of having a normal blood sugar level. In pregnancy optimal diabetic control is considered to equate with a consistent blood sugar 3.5–4.5 mmol/l with 5.5 mmol/l being exceeded only rarely
- **Gestational diabetes mellitus**: GDM describes women who become intolerant of carbohydrate in pregnancy. The cause is usually insulin resistance and/or islet cell insufficiency, although occasionally islet cell failure producing Type 1 (insulin dependent) diabetes will present in pregnancy. Diagnosis is made by glucose tolerance testing (GTT) which shows a diabetic pattern. Insulin is required
- **gestational impaired glucose tolerance**: GIGT describes an abnormal GTT but in less severe form than the frankly diabetic GDM. Dietary modification and/or insulin may be required
- **potential diabetics** are women who have a close family history of diabetes mellitus, a previous large-for-dates baby or who are massively overweight. The term has significance in screening for women at risk of GDM of GIGT. Sadly, it is poorly predicative with low sensitivity and specificity

What is so bad about diabetes in pregnancy?

- **deterioration of maternal condition** in insulin dependent diabetes mellitus (IDDM) can occur. Of particular worry are women with retinopathy and nephropathy. Women with

IDDM planning pregnancy should have any retinal disease attended to prior to conception. Women with significant renal impairment may be advised to consider not becoming pregnant (a creatinine clearance rate of at least 40 ml/min appears to be required for any hope of good maternal and fetal outcome)

- **fetal abnormality** is considerably higher in women with poor glycaemic control around conception and in the first few weeks of pregnancy. Quoted fetal anomaly rates vary from under 3% to nearly 12% depending upon population and method of observation. Cardiac and neural tube defects are more common. Caudal regression is peculiar to diabetics and describes hypotrophy or absence of caudal structures. Fetal anomaly is significantly reduced by achieving pre-pregnancy euglycaemia. There are worries that more subtle anomalies may not present for some years, eg. brain dysfunction manifesting as behavioural problems

- **jaundice** is more common in macrosomic babies. It may be related to polycythaemia

- **macrosomia** describes the polycythaemia, adiposity and organomegally that produce large-for-dates babies in hyperglycaemic women. The cause is fetal hyperinsulinism induced by the facilitated transport of excess amounts of glucose from the maternal circulation. The head and brain are not overgrown making the baby asymmetrical. Such big babies are at increased risk of birth asphyxia and trauma, especially shoulder dystocia

- **miscarriage** is more common in diabetic women

- **neonatal hypoglycaemia** in the first few hours after delivery is common in macrosomic babies and where maternal glycaemic control was poor. Withdrawal of maternal glucose at delivery is not followed by an immediate reduction in fetal insulin levels. Intravenous glucose infusion may be required. If unrecognised, it can cause neonatal brain damage

- **oral hypoglycaemic agents**: until recently these agents have been considered contraindicated in pregnancy. However, recent evidence suggests that they may be safe. Some gynaecologists are successfully treating PCOS with metformin knowing that treatment may overlap early pregnancy.

- **perinatal mortality** in poorly controlled GDM/IDDM is high. If control is optimal and fetal anomaly excluded PNMRs are equivalent to the general population. Of particular concern however, has been the high incidence of 'unexplained' intrauterine deaths at term in diabetics

- **respiratory distress syndrome** is more common in GDM/IDDM pregnancies. The production of surfactant appears to be deficient in macrosomic babies. This was compounded previously by the policy of pre-term delivery to avoid the risk of intrauterine death

- **traumatic delivery** contributes to morbidity and mortality. Shoulder dystocia is the most feared event

Clinical situations

- **diabetic women who plan to become pregnant** should have a detailed workup with major input from their diabetologist. Those with nephropathy and retinopathy are most vulnerable. In women with poor renal function the advisability of becoming pregnant at all will need to be addressed. Retinal screening and, if necessary, treatment should be offered preconceptually. Obviously the other preconceptual questions will need to be covered (rubella status, folic acid supplements etc, see *Chapter 4*). Those taking oral hypoglycaemics will need to transfer to insulin. Those on insulin will need to have the insulin type and blood sugar/injection regimes attended to. Women who are overweight will be helped and encouraged to lose weight. It is essential to push the message of preconceptual workup to teenage girls with diabetes in order to avoid unplanned pregnancies and poor glycaemic control in early pregnancy

- **diabetic women who present pregnant** have a problem. The opportunities to reduce fetal abnormality at the time of organogenesis will have been missed, although the same principles discussed above apply. Euglycaemia is essential and if necessary a period of time as an in-patient may be necessary. Emotional lability and stress can disturb glycaemic control so lifestyle during the pregnancy should be discussed (especially working arrangements)

- **women who become diabetic during pregnancy** are more likely to be encountered in the primary care setting than those with IDDM. Screening is traditionally offered by random urinalysis. This has been shown to be poorly predictive in terms of sensitivity and specificity. Most women have glycosuria at some stage in pregnancy and many women with GIGT will never have glycosuria detected. Offering a GTT to 'potential diabetics' is similarly poor as a screening test. Less than half of the women who develop GDM will have been spotted as potential diabetics. There is no uniform approach although modifications of the GTT have been shown to be useful (75 g oral glucose load followed by a one hour blood sugar). GDM can be diagnosed by finding a fasting sugar ≥ 8 mmol/l, or after a 75g glucose load a one hour glucose >10.5 mmol/l, or a two hour level >9 mmol/l. This is generally done between 26–30 weeks gestation. Another method is to screen thoroughly those with risk factors **and** those with a one hour post 50G load level ≥ 7.8 mmol/l at booking for antenatal care. Be guided by your local obstetrician with an interest in diabetes.

Women with GDM/GIGT in one pregnancy should be actively screened for it in future pregnancies. It is usual to perform a GTT 6–12 weeks postpartum in women with GDM/GIGT. Attention to diet and weight may reduce their future risk of developing non-gestational diabetes mellitus

Amniotic fluid anomaly

The amniotic fluid or liquor is a placental secretion in early pregnancy but the fetus contributes increasingly as pregnancy progresses. The fetus contributes to the fluid via its kidneys as urine and via the lungs as transudated fluid. The fetus also drinks the fluid during pregnancy. An excess of liquor is termed hydramnios or polyhydramnios and its deficiency, oligohydramnios. Diagnosis can be made subjectively or semi-objectively by ultrasonic scanning and measurement of depth of fluid pools. A relative lack of liquor is taken as a sign of poor placental function or fetal compromise.

Hydramnios/polyhydramnios

Hydramnios/polyhydramnios should prompt further investigation. Hydramnios causes maternal discomfort, increases the risk of premature rupture of membranes and preterm labour. Sudden and rapid release of liquor at membrane rupture can provoke placental abruption. The particular diagnoses that should be considered include:

- **fetal gastrointestinal atresia**, eg. tracheo-oesophageal fistula, duodenal atresia
- **hydrops fetalis**: describes fetal dropsy or oedema. It can develop, for example, after maternal parvovirus induced anaemia or in Rhesus sensitised pregnancies

- **twin/twin transfusion syndrome** especially if severe and of sudden onset in the second trimester in a twin pregnancy
- **monozygotic twin pregnancy**
- **maternal diabetes** is associated with hydramnios, perhaps resulting from fetal polyuria
- **maternal hypertension** is linked to hydramnios. If hydramnios develops in a singleton and apparently normal fetus pregnancy, there is a significant risk of hypertension or pre-eclampsia developing

Oligohydramnios

Oligohydramnios is a non-specific sign of poor fetal nutrition or condition. The following should be considered:

- **fetal anomaly** especially renal agenesis
- **fetal growth retardation:** the link may be poor placental nourishment of the fetus and poor placental liquor production. Recent work suggests that IUGR leads to decreased fetal renal blood flow and, as a result, urine output is low resulting in oligohydramnios

Anaemia

Because anaemia is diagnosed far more frequently than it actually occurs, over-treatment in both primary and secondary care is the norm. Iron, however, is a drug with toxic side-effects and can cause death when taken inadvertently by toddlers. The source of confusion is the assumption that non-pregnant haematological indices equate with those in pregnancy. In pregnancy, haemoglobin drops as the red cell mass increases because the plasma volume increase is even greater (physiological haemodilution). Similarly, ferritin is not helpful in pregnancy. Apart from multiple gestation and a few uncommon medical conditions there is no place for 'routine iron therapy' in pregnancy (*Drug and Therapeutics Bulletin*, 1995). There is, however, a place for iron supplements in iron deficiency. To diagnose iron deficiency an early pregnancy or pre-pregnancy FBC is helpful for comparative purposes. Defining parameters for iron deficiency are listed in *Table 6.1*.

Table 6.1: Iron deficiency in pregnancy: definitions

• MCV <82fl
• MCV drop by ≥6fl whatever the previous MCV or Hb
• Hb ó10.5 (empirical and arguably too high)

(Drug Ther Bull, 1995)

GPs should be alert to the possibility of macrocytic change masking iron deficiency, to haemoglobinopathy-induced microcytosis or when treating women with low but physiological Hbs. There is evidence that iron treatment in the absence of deficiency leads to increased blood viscosity and reduces perfusion of the placental bed. Steer advises that GPs should take particular note of the absence of the haemodilution response. The lowest birth weights in his study were seen in women whose Hbs stayed above 14.5 g. Highest birth weights were seen in women whose lowest Hb was 8.5–9.5 g/dl (Steer *et al*, 1995).

Iron: prescribing notes

- Iron is a drug. Can you justify its prescription bearing in mind the data above on the diagnosis of iron deficiency and physiological haemodilution?

- Intolerance to iron preparations is common. Choosing a lower dose preparation or taking fewer doses is advisable. Beware! the milligram dose and the iron content are not the same so perhaps choose a preparation with a lower 'iron content'. See *Table 6.2*

- Modified release preparations carry iron past the first part of the duodenum. Absorption is therefore reduced. This may be the reason they are tolerated better. Why not choose a lower iron content preparation instead?

- Caution in prescribing for women with inflammatory bowel disease and intestinal stricture, especially with m/r preparations

- The average net consequence of pregnancy in iron terms to the mother is just 600 mg, which is equivalent to just 2 mg per day

Table 6.2: The iron content of different iron salts

Iron salt	Iron Content per 100 g
sulphate (dried	32.5 mg
fumarate	32.5 mg
sulphate	20.0 mg
gluconate	12.0 mg

Iron preparations are listed in *Tables 6.3 and 6.4.*

Table 6.3: BNF listed iron preparations

Iron salt	Presentation	Dose	Iron content	Formulation
sulphate	tab tab m/r # tab m/r mixture	200 mg 325 mg 160 mg 60mg/5 ml	65 mg 105 mg 50 mg	non-proprietary Ferrograd Slow-Fe ferrous sulphate oral solution paediatric BP
fumarate	tab tab cap syrup syrup	322 mg 200 mg 305 mg 140 mg/5 ml 140 mg/5 ml	100 mg 65 mg 100 mg 45 mg 45 mg	Fersaday Fersamal Galfer Fersamal Galfer
gluconate	tab	300 mg	35 mg	non-proprietary
glycine sulphate	syrup	141 mg/5ml	25 mg/5 ml	Plesmet
PIC	elixir		100 mg/5 ml	Niferex **
federate	elixir	190 mg/5 ml	27.5 mg/5 ml	Sytron

Principal sources: *MIMS*, November 1999; *BNF* **38**, September 1999

Notes:
*	also contains ascorbic acid
**	NHS = 240ml pack only
#	contains dried ferrous sulphate
FAS	ferrous ammonium citrate
PIC	polysaccharide-iron complex
M/R	modified release

Table 6.4: *BNF* listed NHS iron and folic acid combination preparations

Iron salt	Presentation	Iron content	Folic acid dose	Formulation
sulphate	tab#	105 mg	350 mcg	Ferrograd Folic
	tab m/r	50 mg	400 mcg	Slow-Fe Folic
fumarate	tab	100 mg	350 mcg	Pregaday
	cap	100 mg	350 mcg	Galfer FA
FAS	syrup	80 mg/5 ml	500 mcg	Lexpec with Iron-M

Principal sources: *MIMS* November 1999; *BNF* **38**, September 1999

Notes:
*   also contains ascorbic acid
**   NHS = 240ml pack only
#   contains dried ferrous sulphate
FAS   ferrous ammonium citrate
PIC   polysaccharide-iron complex
M/R   modified release

Bacterial vaginosis

Bacterial vaginosis is implicated in late miscarriage and premature labour. If it is detected the advice of an obstetrician should be sought. Trials are currently underway assessing the value of prophylactic treatment of asymptomatic women in early pregnancy. BV treatments are detailed in *Chapter 1*. Although clindamycin is 'not known to be harmful', metronidazole may be toxic in high dose.

Candidiasis

Candidiasis is common, occurring between 2–10 times more frequently than in non-pregnant women, as does asymptomatic carriage, which rises from 10% in the first to 50% in the third trimester. Candidiasis is also more difficult to eradicate than in non-pregnant women. Azoles (eg. clotimazole) are more effective than nystatin. The oral azoles (itaconazole and fluconazole are contraindicated in pregnancy). Treatments should be for at least three days but do not need to be longer than seven. See tables of preparations in *Chapter 1*.

Caval compression

Caval compression occurs when the weight of the gravid uterus is allowed to flop back onto the sacral promontory, compressing the inferior *vena cava*. Aortic compression is also possible. It is one of the few situations where fainting can be exacerbated by lying down. Caval compression reduces venous return and rapidly decreases cardiac output: 'I feel faint when I lie down doctor'. The way to avoid the problem is to ensure that heavily pregnant women lie to one side when horizontal. The usual measure employed to ensure this in antenatal clinics or, indeed, during Caesarean section, is to place a wedge under the loin of the woman, tipping her slightly and displacing the uterus laterally, away from the *vena cava*.

Constipation

Constipation is complained of in 85% of primigravid pregnancies. It is more common in those with a pre-existing disposition. Initial measures include the addition of fibre and bran to the diet and an increase in fluid intake is essential. The next steps are the addition of bulking agents followed by stool softeners. Irritants are the final medical resort before consideration of secondary care advice or enemas.

- **bulking agents**: bran, ispaghula husk, methylcellulose and stercula are *BNF* listed. These agents are inert and cause few side-effects
- **stool softeners**: lactitol, lactulose are *BNF* listed. These agents are inert and cause few side-effects
- **irritant laxatives**: bisacodyl, danthron, docusate, glycerol (suppositories) and senna are *BNF* listed. These agents are absorbed and cross the placenta, but can be used in resistant cases
- **saline cathartics** containing magnesium or potassium salts are contraindicated in pregnancy. Electrolyte disturbance is a hazard
- **mineral oil lubricants** are contraindicated in pregnancy. They can reduce vitamin absorption and cause perineal pruritis

Cramps

Cramps occur in around half of all pregnancies. They are mainly nocturnal and respond to massage and stretching. Treatments with calcium, vitamin D and sodium have shown variable results in many poorly organised trials. These treatments are not without hazard. Simple leg stretches and massage are said to be helpful, posing no threat to the pregnancy.

Cytomegalovirus infection

Cytomegalovirus infection (CMV) is the commonest viral infection acquired in pregnancy. CMV is unusual as it can cause recurrent infection. Both primary and recurrent infections can cause fetal infection, although only primary infection gives a significant maternal illness (resembling glandular fever). Maternal CMV is followed by transplacental infection in around one third of cases. Not every infected fetus develops sequelae. Only infection in the first half of pregnancy is likely to result in a congenital CMV syndrome. The features are sensory-neural deafness, mental retardation, chorioretinitis. There is no specific treatment. Although background seropositivity is higher in women from lower socio-economic backgrounds, congenital infection is also more common. The explanation may be that exposure to toddlers and babies who may shed virus in the urine may be higher (Stagno, 1986). Fetal infection through reactivated CMV infection in HIV positive women has been documented. There is no indication for routine screening for CMV.

Pregnant healthcare workers should be aware of the higher risk of exposure to CMV when in contact with HIV positive patients who have a particular vulnerability to this virus.

Dyspepsia

Heartburn (dyspepsia) is complained of by two-thirds of women during pregnancy. It is related to eating and posture, especially stooping and lying. First line advice is to take smaller meals and avoid eating for several hours before retiring at night. Propping up the head of the bed is said to help, as are extra pillows. The avoidance of fatty and spicy foods helps others. All the antacids have similar effects although gel formulations give better results than liquids. Excessive use of antacids can lead to metabolic disorder; sodium salts can cause sodium overload and are best avoided, magnesium salts can cause diarrhoea, calcium salts can cause hypercalcaemia, impairment of renal function and gastric hypersecretion. Aluminium salts can lead to phosphate depletion. The effect of medication is enhanced if it is palatable. Proprietary antacids are best avoided as many contain other ingredients (antispasmodics, anticholinergics). Curiously, for more severe or persistent problems diluted hydrochloric acid has been used to good effect. 'Dilute HCl BP' should be diluted further (0.1 ml in 10 ml of water, a hundred-fold dilution) to pH2. It may be that it works by neutralising refluxed duodenal contents in the stomach.

For more severe symptoms, the involvement of a gastroenterologist may be considered. Cimetidine and misoprostol are contraindicated in pregnancy. Ranitidine and omeprazol have been used without evidence of fetal compromise.

Genital infection

Genital infection in pregnancy is contiguous with genital infection in women in their fertile years.

- *candidal infection* is far more common in pregnancy and is discussed above and in *Chapter 1*, specific treatments are also listed
- *bacterial vaginosis* is discussed above and in *Chapter 1*
- *β haemolytic streptococci* is discussed below. Premature rupture of the membranes and pre-term labour are linked to this infection. Catastrophic neonatal infection is the principal anxiety
- *herpes virus* (simplex and zoster) are discussed below
- *human papilloma virus*, genital: wart virus can be picked up in labour and delivery by the fetus. Seek specialist advice

- **sexually transmissible disease** always requires specialist advice and help in pregnancy as it does in the non-pregnant condition. The active involvement of the specialist nursing services in GUMed departments is desirable

β haemolytic streptoccocal infection

β haemolytic streptoccocal infection can be catastrophic in the fetus and neonate. This group of organisms was classically responsible for the puerperal sepsis so common in the last century. There is a strong association with premature and prolonged rupture of the fetal membranes, intrapartum fever and puerperal sepsis. In any of these circumstances bacteriological investigation should be instigated. It can cause fetal/neonatal respiratory distress syndrome and septic shock which can be of rapid onset and overwhelming in its severity. The carriage rate in pregnant women is quoted as 12%; however, antepartum screening and treatment of asymptomatic carriers is rapidly followed by recolonisation. Intrapartum prophyaxis after identification of its presence using a rapid diagnostic testing method has been shown to be of great benefit. Guidelines on screening for β haemolytic streptoccocal infection during late pregnancy will be appearing soon, but will have greater relevance to intrapartum physicians. Risk factors that may prompt investigation include:

- pre-term labour
- premature rupture of membranes
- prolonged rupture of membranes
- previously affected neonate.

Haemorrhage (antepartum)

Bleeding in pregnancy is never normal although it does not necessarily imply serious pathology. Antepartum haemorrhage (APH) was previously defined as genital tract bleeding after twenty-eight weeks gestation. With improving fetal outcome at earlier gestations, most units now treat bleeding after twenty weeks as APH. Although *placenta praevia* and abruption are the most important causes of APH they are the cause of a minority of cases. There is, however, no room for complacency as each triennial Maternal Mortality Report will testify. Urgent hospitalisation is almost always indicated. In anything other than minor bleeds the only primary care options are siting an intravenous line and taking blood for cross-matching while awaiting the arrival of the ambulance. A classification of APH follows but do not fail to read the clinical points on the place of vaginal examination in APH (almost none) and Rhesus complication of APH.

Causes

placenta praevia

Placenta praevia or 'inevitable haemorrhage' produces painless vaginal bleeding. Low implantation may result in the placenta enroaching onto the lower uterine segment or in its more florid forms covering the internal cervical os. Warning bleeds may occur before catastrophic haemorrhage. Diagnosis should be made by obstetricians on ultrasound scanning or magnetic resonance imaging. Praevia is said to be more common in older and multiparous women. It is more common in multiple gestation and in women with previous uterine trauma (Caesarean section, D&C, previous evacuation of retained products of conception). There is no primary care management of bleeding from placenta praevia but women with an ultrasonically demonstrated low placenta may be managed at home by obstetricians.

abruptio placentae

Abruptio placentae or 'accidental haemorrhage' describes retroplacental bleeding. A clot may form between the placenta and the myometrium. The stripping of the placenta from the uterus by clot results in fetal hypoxia and, if severe, maternal collapse. There is an association with a maternal age and parity, rapid loss of amniotic fluid when the membranes rupture, multiple pregnancy and cocaine abuse. Hypertension is associated but whether by cause or effect is unclear. Poor placentation is cited as a cause as is chorioamnionitis. Abruption may result from trauma, the classic case being road traffic accident. Seat belt injury has been reported. Consider admission of all women who are pregnant after RTA, as abruption can develop after several hours after quite trivial decelerations. The main symptom is uterine pain. External bleeding may not occur even in severe cases. The principal signs are increased uterine tone, uterine tenderness, difficulty feeling fetal parts and hearing the fetal heart. In severe cases, maternal shock develops and can lead to disseminated intravascular coagulation.

marginal haemorrhage

Marginal haemorrhage may occur when the rim of the placenta lifts itself off the myometrium. Some bleeding will occur and may reveal itself vaginally. Unlike abruption, marginal haemorrhage is not necessarily a progressive condition.

vasa praevia

Vasa praevia describes the presence of fetal blood vessels within the portion of the membranes that cover the cervical os. For it to occur there must be a velamentous insertion of the umbilical cord, ie. attachment to the membranes rather than to the placenta, and the umbilical vessels must course across the membranes over the internal os before gaining the placenta. It is rare, usually presents in labour after rupture of the membranes and is very difficult to diagnose. It causes light painless vaginal bleeding without maternal symptoms but with fetal distress. Diagnosis requires a high index of suspicion and the demonstration that the blood is fetal and not maternal.

local causes of APH

Local causes of APH are common and will usually present to the primary care professionals. The most common result from minor abrasions of the lower genital tract, especially the cervix, perhaps following sexual intercourse. Cervical cancer is a rare but important cause. Primary care professionals should never be lulled into complacency as massive haemorrhage from a *placenta praevia* may be preceded by light warning bleeds.

feto-maternal haemorrhage

Feto-maternal haemorrhage is very difficult to diagnose. Small shuts may be suspected only when a Rhesus negative woman develops anti-D antibodies. Larger bleeds can exsanguinate the fetus. The only symptom may be reduced fetal movement and the only sign fetal heart rate anomalies. Diagnosis is clinched when Kliehaur testing demonstrates fetal erythrocytes in the maternal circulation.

Clinical points

vaginal examination in APH

Don't! *Placenta pracvia* can only be excluded by ultrasound examination. Inadvertent digital examination can provoke fatal maternal bleeding. Vaginal examination by an experienced obstetrician in an operating theatre prepared to perform immediate Caesarean section on an anaesthetised cross-matched woman is permissible.

Rhesus negative women

Rhesus negative women can be iso-immunised by APH. Feto-maternal transfusion of even trivial amounts can result in maternal antibody formation. Kliehaur testing can identify women who need anti-D immunoglobulin and quantification of the transfusion will suggest the dose that is required. Knowledge of the maternal Rhesus status is mandatory in cases of APH as, indeed, it is in cases of threatened miscarriage. Unrevealed minor APH resulting in feto-maternal bleeding remains a cause of occult Rhesus sensitisation that is difficult to manage. Some countries run programmes screening Rhesus negative women frequently through pregnancy in an attempt to reduce the problem. Supplies of the immunoglobulin and its price are a constraint in the UK.

Haemorrhage (postpartum)

Postpartum haemorrhage (PPH) is defined in two ways: primary and secondary.

Primary PPH

Primary PPH is defined as blood loss in excess of 500 ml in the first twenty-four hours after delivery. Blood loss >1L is considered severe. Primary PPH occurring in a domiciliary setting should prompt urgent arrangements for transfer to an obstetric unit. It should be remembered that hypotension is a late sign in severe PPH; early signs of decompensation include tachycardia >100/bpm and tachypnoea >15/min. Risk factors for PPH include:

- pregnancy-induced hypertension and pre-eclampsia
- arrest of decent of presenting part
- prolonged third stage of labour
- episiotomy and genital tract trauma
- previous PPH
- multiple gestation
- bleeding tendency: this may be an acute problem associated with, for example, pre-eclampsia.

primiparity and augmentation of labour

Primiparity and augmentation of labour do not appear to be significant factors when other risk factors are controlled, for example, pregnancy induced hypertension.

management of the third stage

The management of the third stage is important. Active management involves administration of an oxytocic with delivery of the anterior shoulder and controlled cord traction after delivery (NB oxytocics are delayed until the last fetus is delivered in multiple gestation). Physiological management avoids the use of oxytocics unless clinically indicated and allows spontaneous expulsion of the placenta. Although active management is associated with more manual removals of placentae, the PPH rate is significantly lower (6% vs 18%) as is the incidence of severe PPH. The requirement for blood transfusion and need for intravenous oxytocics are also lower.

oxytocics

Oxytocics in the form of ergometrine had a massive impact on morbidity and mortality when introduced in the 1930s. Ergometrine is used only in emergencies. Oxytocin is used when ergometrine is contraindicated. Syntometrine is the usual routine third stage oxytocic. See *Table 6.5.*

Table 6.5: *BNF* listed oxytocics

Drug	Formulation	Notes
Syntometrine 1 ml amp	oxytocin 5 u/ml, ergometrine 500 mcg/ml	The usual primary care oxytocic. Must be kept out of light and <22°C. Shelf life — 3 months max. See ergometrine cautions and contraindications. Give im or slow iv if high risk situation exists
ergometrine 1 ml amp	500 mcg/ml (also available as tablets; see 2° PPH)	Frequently induces nausea or vomiting. Caution in hypertension, cardiac disease, renal and hepatic impairment. Contraindicated in pre-eclampsia, pulmonary impairment or if any of the cautions are severe; im or slow iv if the situation warrants
oxytocin 1 ml amp	5 u/ml, 10 u/ml	Slow iv injection of 5u in cases where ergometrine is contraindicated

Secondary PPH

Secondary PPH is defined as abnormal bleeding after the first twenty-four hours but before six weeks. The majority of cases occur in the second week and so most women with 2° PPH will present to primary care professionals. Secondary PPH is usually caused by infection, retained products of conception or both. Minor bleeding in a woman who is well may be managed at home with antibiotics for presumed infection. Co-amoxiclav or amoxicillin/metronidazole are recommended. Bleeding as heavy as a period or accompanied by clots, or where the woman is unwell, socially isolated or anaemic should be managed in hospital (the baby should be admitted too). Oral ergometrine is listed in the *BNF.* The dose is 500 mcg tds for three days and the cautions and contraindications are the same as for parenteral use. They should not be used in the presence of retained products of conception.

Heartburn

See above, dyspepsia.

HELLP syndrome

HELLP syndrome does not have precise diagnostic criteria. The acronym stands for haemolysis, elevated liver enzymes and low platelets. There is considerable overlap with HELLP and pre-eclampsia. Severity ranges from mild to fulminating which has a high mortality. The syndrome presents most commonly in the third trimester and is usually associated with raised blood pressure; it occasionally presents after delivery. No primary care options available.

Hepatitis B

Of the known causes of cancer, only tobacco ranks higher than the hepatitis B virus world-wide. In areas of high prevalence it has been shown to be worthwhile to screen all pregnant women for HB surface antigen and to offer the babies of HBsAg positive women immunoprophylaxis at birth. In the UK screening is not uniform but is offered to most women from high risk groups (see *Table 6.6*). Only low level transplacental passage of virus occurs. However, maternal anti-hepatitis antibodies do cross the placenta. These shield the fetus and account for the observation that most vertical infection occurs around the time of delivery. Immediate passive immunisation of the baby with hepatitis B immunoglobulin (not γ globulin) provides good protection. HB antigen positive mothers should be encouraged to nurse and comfort their babies, and breast feed them too if this is desired, but only if immunoprophylaxis has been commenced. Unlike HIV, Caesarean section has not been shown to reduce virus transmission to the baby. Horizontal transmission to the child after delivery is also reduced by immunoprophylaxis at birth.

Herpes simplex

Herpes simplex can be transmitted to the neonate and may be severe. Careful hygiene is essential. Maternal genital herpetic infection should be managed by obstetricians and GU medicine specialists in concert.

Table 6.6: Risk factors for Hepatitis B antigen positive status

Risk factors used to screen selectively women for HBsAg
● women from high risk areas of the world *(this includes first and second generation immigrants)
● women with a history of liver disorder
● women with potential occupational exposure
● women with partners from high risk areas *
● women donors rejected by the blood transfusion service
● women who have had multiple blood transfusions
● women with tattoos inflicted while in a high risk area *
● women with impaired immunity
● women with a history of sexually transmitted disease
● intravenous drug abusers and/or sexual partners of such
● close household contacts with people from high risk groups (eg. bisexual men)

* Asia, Africa, Middle East, Haiti and the Mediterranean countries

Human immunodeficiency virus (HIV)

HIV targets the CD4 T lymphocyte and presently infects four per thousand adults world-wide. By the turn of the century it is estimated that the world-wide burden on humanity will be 30–40 million infected people of whom 4–8 million will be children. In the United States HIV related disease is the leading cause of mortality during pregnancy. A thorough discussion of HIV/AIDS and primary care management during and after pregnancy is not pursued here. A good presentation of the data can be found in '*Women and HIV*' (Gupta, 1997). New data is being published daily. There are several reasons why awareness of HIV seropositive status is beneficial to prospective mothers (see *Table 6.7*).

Table 6.7: Benefits of knowledge of HIV antibody status

Benefits of knowledge of HIV positive status
● enables choice on whether embarking on pregnancy is desirable
● enables consideration of termination of pregnancy to be made
● can lead to protection of HIV negative partner(s)
● can reduce risk of vertical transmission
● allows women to adopt a healthier lifestyle
● allows anti-retroviral therapy to be commenced
● allows HIV related disorders to be recognised and treated promptly
● allows prompt recognition and treatment of infection in the baby/child

Key issues

screening

Screening for HIV status should be offered to all pregnant women where the community seroprevalence rates are high. Selective screening should be offered otherwise (*Table 6.8*). Selection requires identification of women with risk factors for HIV positive status. Testing those identified risks stigmatises the woman but may be the lesser of two evils. As with all screening tests it can only be offered if some benefit may accrue. Pre-pregnancy testing is preferable. Screening should be offered only by those with appropriate training on the issues, particularly on counselling women whatever the result of the test. As the level of heterosexual transmission in a community rises, universal rather than selective screening, becomes more worthwhile (as it now is in some London antenatal clinics).

Table 6.8: Higher risk groups for positive HIV status

Criteria for selective HIV testing *
● illicit drug users
● sexual partners of men who have had sex with other men
● sexual partners of drug users (especially intravenous drug use since 1977)
● sexual partners of men living in Africa (excluding Mediterranean countries)
● sexual partners of haemophiliacs
● sex industry workers (prostitutes)

* testing must be appropriate for the population being screened

effects of HIV on pregnancy

Effects of HIV on pregnancy are not known for sure. Reporting bias probably promoted an over pessimistic view earlier, but the maternal consequence may be a higher than usual predilection for infection. See below for fetal effects.

effects of pregnancy on HIV disease

Progression rates are probably unaffected. CD4 counts naturally drop in pregnancy. The significance of this in HIV infected women is not known.

presentation of HIV in pregnancy

Primary infection or first development of symptomatic disease tends to be innocuous. In women at particular risk of HIV seropositivity tiredness, anorexia, weight loss, breathlessness, cough, diarrhoea or dyspepsia should ring bells and prompt moves to discussing HIV testing.

vertical transmission risk

Vertical transmission risk from an HIV positive mother to her baby is around one in seven. Pre-term delivery may increase it. Primary infection during pregnancy with a high viraemia appears to increase the fetal risk; perhaps as high as one in three. The consensus is that most transmissions occur around the time of delivery. Caesarean delivery appears to reduce the transmission rate. Placental damage, eg. chorioamnionitis increases the risk. A registry of exposed twins is expected to give useful data in the future.

breast feeding and the HIV positive woman

The chance of acquiring the HIV virus is higher in breast fed children. The longer the duration of breast feeding the greater the risk of contracting the virus. In developed countries with access to safe formula feeds, breast feeding should be discouraged. In developing countries where hygiene may be difficult and reliable supplies of quality milk feeds unlikely then lactation promotion is preferable. Colostrum appears to be more hazardous than milk from established lactators.

CMV and toxoplasmosis

CMV and toxoplasmosis should be screened for in HIV positive women (as should hepatitis B, syphilis, gonorrhoea, chlamydia and cervical dysplasia). Both infections can re-activate in women with HIV. Primary, but not reactivated toxoplasmosis is thought to pose fetal risk. However, primary and reactivated CMV is a definite source of risk to the fetus. CMV may also be a hazard to pregnant attendants of HIV positive people.

management of HIV infected women during and after pregnancy

Anti-retroviral therapy with azidothymidine (AZT, Zidovudine) appears to confer benefit and may reduce vertical transmission. The question of prophylactic use of AZT and therapies against pneumocystis carenii are for secondary care specialists in the field. Currently AZT in pregnancy, Caesarean section delivery and avoidance of breast feeding appear to be the best choices for the baby. New data is coming along constantly.

needlestick injury

Needlestick injury to you or anyone else resulting in the inoculation of HIV positive blood carries a risk of seroconversion (assuming you have not got it already) of 0.38% according to one large study of over two thousand cases.

Hyperemesis gravidarum

Hyperemesis gravidarum lies at one end of the emesis spectrum. Dehydration, ketosis, ketonuria requiring admission and intravenous therapy is uncommon. However, nausea is experienced by 70% of pregnant women and vomiting by around 50%. It is usually fairly transient and although unpleasant is rarely clinically significant. It is more frequent in primigravidas, the young and the overweight. It is also a sign of multiple gestation and trophoblastic disease. Of a little comfort is the knowledge that nausea and vomiting are far less common in ectopic pregnancy and in pregnancies doomed to miscarry. Nausea and vomiting usually respond to taking smaller more frequent meals and the avoidance of cooking smells and stale odours. Drugs can help too. The placebo effect is high and uncontrolled trials have found many drugs to be apparently effective. This is common in self-limiting conditions and uncontrolled trials. Simple anti-histamines however, are traditionally used and are considered safe (eg. promethazine theoclate). Cyclizine, meclozine and dipheniramine are commonly used but there have been suggestions of a link between their use and facial clefts in the fetus. Antihistamines are more effective than placebos. They can however sedate and cause blurred vision, so caution against driving. The most effective drug, Debendox (doxylamine succinate and pyridoxine), is no longer marketed. The manufacturers found the legal costs of defence against spurious claims of teratogenesis overwhelming. Such drugs can be classed as 'litogens'. ***Astemazole (Hismanal) is contraindicated in pregnancy and lactation.*** Phenothiazine related anti-emetics are best avoided as they can cause extra-pyramidal effects, jaundice and, in early pregnancy, are considered embryotoxic. Vitamin B_6 (pyridoxine) and metoclopramide has been shown to be of some benefit. A recent report has found that severe intractable hyperemesis gravidarum may respond dramatically to high dose corticosteroids. Some women have found the acupressure over the neugian point proximal to the anterior wrist crease using 'sea bands' of help. There may be a link between maternal carriage of Helicobacter Pylori and hyperemesis gravidarum. It is postulated that early pregnancy changes in gastric fluid pH may allow asymptomatic *H pylori* organisms to flourish (Frigo P, 1998).

Hypertension in pregnancy

Hypertension in pregnancy must be rigorously distinguished from pre-eclampsia. Hypertension can pre-date the pregnancy (and is known as chronic hypertension), or it may occur *de novo* during pregnancy — pregnancy-induced hypertension (PIH). New hypertension in the second half of pregnancy is usually a sign of pre-eclampsia which is fully discussed under pre-eclampsia/eclampsia.

Pre-conceptual attention to teratogenic potential of medication in known hypertensives is advisable as is testing for the presence of renal damage. If doubts exist the opinions and help of an obstetrician with a particular interest should be sought.

Accepted definitions of PIH are finding a raised blood pressure after 20 weeks' gestation in a woman known previously to be normotensive. Chronic hypertension may be defined as:

- phase V diastolic $\geq$110mmHg
- phase V diastolic $\geq$90mmHg on two occasions at least 4 hours apart
- finding a sustained diastolic blood pressure 15mmHg >early pregnancy level
- finding a sustained systolic blood pressure 30mmHg >early pregnancy level

Infantile colic

Infantile colic is common, transient and self-limiting. It can, however, be extremely distressing for the new parents. It typically afflicts healthy, thriving babies who cry persistently, perhaps drawing their legs up, passing wind p.r., belching and occasionally with abdominal distension. As is typical in self-limiting conditions, all treatments appear to work. Gripe waters are often used and no longer contain ethanol in their formulation. The primary care professional's input falls into five categories:

- ***excluding other conditions***
- ***parental reassurance and support***

- ***dietary manipulations***: some infants appear to benefit from a change from cow's milk formulas to soya milk. It needs to be stressed to the parents that this does not imply allergy and milk can be re-introduced later on without anxiety
- ***drug treatment*** involves giving activated dimethacone. The *BNF* lists Infacol (activated dimethacone) 40 mg/ml dispensed in 50 ml packs. Usual dose is 0.5 ml before feeds. The *Drug and Therapeutics Bulletin* described Infracol as a 'non-toxic, non-absorbed agent that reduces mucus surface tension allowing gas bubbles to coalesce' which facilitates their passage orally or p.r.
- ***breast feeding***: there is evidence that the watery fore-milk which is more sugary than the hind-milk can be fermented releasing gas. If the infant is moved from one breast to the other before the let down of hind-mild she/he will not get the ideal mix of the two. The excess fore-milk may then promote the development of gas

A recent review of the various interventions found, benefit with short term substitution of cows milk formulas with hypoallergenic or soya based milks and certain parental behavioural modifications. Dicyclomine and simethicone were not shown to be beneficial (Lucassen P, 1998).

Jaundice

Jaundice can occur incidentally or be caused by the pregnancy itself. There are several conditions that must be considered in any case of jaundice in pregnancy:

- ***incidental causes of jaundice*** include viral hepatitis, auto-immune hepatitis, cholelithiasis
- ***intrahepatic cholestasis of pregnancy*** occurs to some degree in up to 2% of all pregnancies. The cardinal features are mild jaundice and pruritis which may be severe. Associated features include tiredness, malaise, anorexia, mild abdominal pain and signs of mild obstructive jaundice. Sufferers may relapse if given the combined oral contraceptive pill. The cause appears to be oestrogen which impairs the function of the hepatocyte. Resolution occurs after delivery:
  - treatment of the pruritis is symptomatic; cholestyramine is only moderately effective
  - Vitamin K supplementation is required by the mother and should be given to the baby immediately after delivery. This reduces post-partum haemorrhage and haemorrhagic disease of the new-born
  - careful fetal monitoring is required as there is an increased incidence of intrauterine death
- ***acute fatty liver of pregnancy*** is a far less common but much more serious problem than cholestasis of pregnancy. It complicates around 1:10,000 pregnancies and has a maternal mortality rate of around 30%. It is commoner in the obese, in twin pregnancies, in the pre-eclamptic and in the presence of a male fetus. It usually presents with symptoms and signs in the third trimester. It is a cause of acute liver failure and consumptive coagulopathy. Symptoms include nausea, vomiting, pruritis, abdominal and back pain. Signs include icterus, features of colitis and pancreatitis and ascites. Tertiary multi-disciplinary care is indicated with urgency
- ***HELLP syndrome*** is discussed above separately.

Listeriosis

Infection with the gram positive rod bacillus *listeria monocytogenes*. Listeriosis is a rare cause of maternal fever and fetal infection (1:30,000 births in 1990). The organism is widely spread in nature being a contaminant of food and animals. The bowel carriage rate is around 20%. It can grow at temperatures as low as 6°C and can resist temperatures as high as 70°C for two minutes. It can cause maternal pyrexia which may be devoid of pathognomonic signs. Maternal myalgia, headache, backache and a flu' like illness are common. It can mimic UTI. Meningoencephalitis may occur. The fetal consequences of infection were classically described as 'granulomatosis infantiseptica'. Septicaemia, jaundice, pneumonia, meningoencephalitis and stillbirth are possibilities. Neonatal infection is severe. Diagnosis is confirmed by blood culture, although only a high index of suspicion in any persistently pyrexial pregnant women will prompt the attendant to perform the diagnostic test in the first place. Blood cultures specifying suspected listeria should be sent on women with an unexplained pyrexia of 48 hours. Avoidance measures include abstaining from paté and soft cheeses during pregnancy and the thorough cooking of all foods, especially chicken. Cook-chill meals should be kept cool until thoroughly cooked and consumed soon after purchase (see CMO communication, 1992).

Nausea

See hyperemesis gravidarum, but always consider that other causes of this symptom/sign may be responsible.

Oedema

Oedema affects half of all pregnancies. It is generally pedal. Pitting and generalised oedema should prompt screening for pre-eclampsia and renal disorder. Diuretics have little place in general and no place in pre-eclampsia where intravascular compartment depletion already exists. The simple measures of exercise, elevation at rest and compression should be advised along with reassurance if more serious disorder is excluded.

Parvovirus B19

Parvovirus B19 is the organism that causes the 'slapped cheek' syndrome in children. Also known as fifth disease and *erythema infectiosum*. Around 40% of the adult population are non-immune. Primary infection produces the characteristic rash and in adults may be associated with an acute but transient arthritis. Only around 10% of fetuses will be infected in an acute maternal illness. Parvovirus infection can cause late miscarriage, premature delivery and, importantly, an acute fetal anaemic crisis. This produces hydrops which may lead to intrauterine fetal death but is detectable ultrasonically. Intrauterine blood transfusion can be lifesaving. If maternal infection is suspected an urgent obstetric opinion is advisable. Infection during the first 24 weeks of gestation is most hazardous.

Perinatal mortality

Perinatal mortality describes the delivery of a stillborn infant or a liveborn infant that fails to survive for one week. It is a crude marker for community health standards. Of much more relevance to primary care professionals are the couples and their families who suffer the tragedy of perinatal bereavement. The Stillbirth and Neonatal Death Society produces an excellent publication which is required reading not only for primary and secondary health care professionals but also has particular advice for civil servants, funeral directors, chaplains etc. (SANDS, 1991).

Perineal care

There is a vast range of preparations that may be applied to the perineum or taken orally after childbirth to relieve perineal discomfort and pain. Unfortunately very little evidence exists that any are of much use. Such trials that have been done find placebos quite good and it is likely that placebos are what these therapies actually are. It behoves the carer to make sure her/his placebos are harmless.

- ***principles of healing***: the perineum is biologically no different from any other portion of the body's surface and as such will recover from bruising, laceration, oedema and infection in the same way. The first question one must ask is therefore 'would I apply the same remedies to other traumatised areas just as enthusiastically?' eg. to a crushed and lacerated hand. Avoidance of compression and pressure, removal of moisture and secretions, prompt treatment of infection, keeping the area cool and dry and patiently allowing time for healing to occur must surely be primary principles. In addition, avoiding discomfort during defecation is important. Codeine-based analgesics can constipate quickly

- ***soothing remedies*** appear to work, but only for a short period of time. Cool baths, Sitz baths, saline baths, warm baths, ice packs etc. all give short term relief. Topical anaesthetic agents also sooth and relieve but again the effects are transient. Topical anaesthetics will sensitise the skin if used repeatedly. Oral analgesics are also useful and common choices begin with paracetamol and range through codeine to ibuprofen. Caution in lactating women and avoidance of constipation are important. Many women find sitting on a ring which avoids pressure on the perineum is helpful

- ***healing remedies*** abound, but trials proving their worth do not. Enkin (1994) lists ultrasonic and electromagnetic therapies in the 'awaiting further evaluation' category

Piles

Piles complicate a large proportion of pregnancies. They commonly produce bleeding, irritation, a mucoid discharge and pain. The mechanism is thought to be a combination of the hormonal effects of pregnancy on the vasculature, compression of pelvic veins by the enlarging pregnancy and the special anatomy of the haemorrhoidal venous drainage system. Nearly half the cases of external haemorrhoids are complicated by internal haemorrhoids. Treatments are aimed at:

- ***excluding other disorders***, eg. malignancy, infection and infestation, inflammatory bowel disease.
- ***ensuring a soft stool*** (or avoiding hard stools) with judicious use of laxatives (see constipation)
- ***avoiding straining*** at stool by avoiding hard and bulky stools
- ***reducing pressure on the haemorrhoidal plexus*** with periods of rest in either a horizontal or slightly head down position. Beware of 'caval compression' by ensuring the woman lies on her side (see caval compression)
- ***applying soothing preparations*** to haemorrhoidal varicosities. There are numerous bland preparations containing bismuth or zinc. Topical heparinoids are said to promote resolution of oedema and bruising. Local anaesthetic agents are formulated into many preparations, but skin sensitisation can develop rapidly
- ***episiotomy and tear repairs*** need to be performed with skill and any subsequent infection treated promptly. See care of the perineum
- ***treating complications*** of haemorrhoids which include infection, thrombosis and prolapse. Very occasionally haemorrhoidectomy may be required during pregnancy. If in doubt, consult the obstetrician or a surgeon with an interest in proctology.

Postpartum collapse

Even a brief survey of the literature on the subject will be characterised by two words: infrequent and terrifying. The four principal causes are discussed below. All require urgent transfer to secondary or tertiary care. All may present during pregnancy as well as in the puerperium.

amniotic fluid embolus

Amniotic fluid embolus describes the rare condition where amniotic fluid and other material from the uterus gains access to the maternal circulation through a breach in the feto-placental circulation. The particulate material may be meconium, vernix caeseosa, fetal squames or other debris. Once in the maternal venous system, embolisation to the pulmonary arterial tree is inevitable. The result is sudden severe dyspnoea, frothy pulmonary oedema and cyanosis. This usually progresses rapidly to unconsciousness, shock and left ventricular failure. Seizures complicate one fifth of cases and disseminated intravascular coagulation is common. The mortality rate approaches 85%. Immediate management is directed to achieving an airway and ventilating if required. Correction of shock with fluids requires some caution because of heart failure. Intensive care in hospital may allow other therapies to be given, eg. digitalisation and measures to cope with coagulopathy.

pulmonary embolus

The risk of thromboembolic disorders is increased in pregnancy and the puerperium. In the four weeks after delivery the risk is around 50 times that in the non-pregnant state. The causes include the hypercoagulable state of pregnancy, compression of the pelvic veins and stasis in the legs, the trauma of delivery (especially Caesarean section) and sepsis. Presentation of PE is the same as in the non-pregnant state. Massive emboli produce dyspnoea, hypotension and cyanosis, and smaller ones are likely to give pain. Management should be urgent and in hospital.

eclampsia

Eclampsia is discussed in the section on Pre-eclampsia/eclampsia.

myocardial infarction

Myocardial infarction is uncommon but serious; over one third of women having an MI in or just after pregnancy die of it. The predispositions are the same as in non-pregnant women but diabetes and obesity are significant factors. Management is the same as in the non-pregnant state.

Post term pregnancy

Post term pregnancy is empirically defined as one continuing beyond the forty-first completed week, that is into and beyond forty-two weeks. The question is whether allowing a pregnancy to continue will risk intrauterine death. The answer is that it possibly could, but against this one must balance the unquantifiable risks of neonatal death that are avoided while the pregnancy continues and the fetus matures. The only proven gain from a policy of induction at term over allowing pregnancy to continue is that meconium staining of the liquor is reduced. It also appears that induction at term is not associated with an increased risk of Caesarean section. Enkin (1994) suggests that only two logical alternatives exist; namely, entering all women with post term pregnancy into a multi-centred randomised trial of induction versus conservative observation or, after informed discussion, following the wishes of the mother. However, most women opt for induction.

Pre-eclampsia/eclampsia

Pre-eclampsia/eclampsia is one of the big five complications of pregnancy. Screening for it is probably **the** principle reason for providing antenatal care. It will complicate 1:20–30 pregnancies in the UK. Death can be caused by pre-eclampsia and its complications and is one of the areas where the primary care professionals feature in each triennial Maternal Mortality Report.

Terminology in hypertensive disorder in pregnancy

- **chronic hypertension** describes pre-existing hypertension. Pre-eclamptic toxaemia (PET) rarely produces signs like a rise in BP in the first half of pregnancy. A raised BP in early pregnancy implies chronic (probably but not necessarily essential) hypertension
- **pregnancy-induced hypertension** describes hypertension first occurring in the second half of pregnancy and resolving after delivery. It may be part of the pre-eclamptic syndrome, but in the absence of other features pre-eclampsia should not be diagnosed. The labels pregnancy-induced hypertension and pre-eclampsia are not interchangeable, although pre-eclampsia may superimpose upon PIH. Precision is important
- **pre-eclampsia** typically is said to present with the symptom triad of hypertension, proteinuria and oedema; would that life were so simple. Pre-eclampsia is rather a pregnancy-induced condition caused by the placenta which can involve the cardiovascular, coagulation, renal, hepatic and nervous systems. Its presenting features are thus legion. There is no sign that is consistently present in pre-eclampsia although proteinuric hypertension is probably the commonest presentation in primary care
- **eclampsia** is a severe neurological complication of pre-eclampsia. It manifests as convulsions and is a form of hypertensive encephalopathy
- **HELLP syndrome** is an uncommon but exceedingly dangerous manifestation of PET. It involves derangement of hepatic and renal function; it is accompanied by a consumptive coagulopathy and a high mortality. It represents one end-point of the pre-eclamptic syndrome

Features of pre-eclampsia

aetiology

Pre-eclampsia appears to be caused by a disorder of placentation. It results in damage to the maternal vascular endothelial system. Its genesis is early in the first trimester, but its symptomatic clinical presentation may be months later; even until the puerperium.

demography

Pre-eclampsia is far more common in primigravidas (x15). Secundigravidas have a far higher incidence if they had pre-eclampsia in their first pregnancy (x10–15). Pre-eclampsia is in fact less common in the obese although such women are more likely to have chronic hypertension. Rather, the small underweight woman is more at risk from pre-eclampsia. Conditions with hyper-placentation are more likely to be complicated by pre-eclampsia, eg. multiple gestation, trophoblastic disease, triploidy, trisomy and hydrops fetalis. Pre-eclampsia is commoner in women with a positive family history of the disorder, in women who have not been exposed to their partners' semenal fluid for long, but it is less common in smokers. Pre-eclampsia appears to be less common in women whose diet is replete with calcium. Whether calcium supplements are protective is not known.

presentation

Presentation is most commonly with proteinuric hypertension. However, it may present more fulminantly with headache, epigastric pain, ascites or pulmonary oedema. Occasionally the first manifestation is as an eclamptic fit. Pre-eclampsia is the commonest cause of nephrotic syndrome in pregnancy.

complications

Complications are legion. Renal and hepatic failure are end points. Encephalopathy, cerebrovascular haemorrhage and particularly cortical blindness are well known. Disseminated intravascular coagulation is particularly ominous. It has been stated that from the first appearance of proteinuria it takes on average three weeks until eclampsia or another urgent requirement to terminate the pregnancy arises.

treatment

Treatment consists of terminating the pregnancy and close observation until it is achieved. Anti-hypertensive therapy will reduce blood pressure for a time but has no effect whatsoever on the underlying pre-eclamptic process. Treatment should be as an in-patient or closely monitored out-patient under secondary care.

Pre-eclamptic toxaemia (PET)

clinical situations

- ***who to screen***: all women should be screened through pregnancy. However primigravidas, those with a personal or family history of the disorder or a predisposition to hyperplacentation (eg. twin pregnancy) should be screened diligently through the second trimester which is generally a time of infrequent monitoring

- ***how to screen***
  - blood-pressure monitoring, preferably in the sitting position
  - urinalysis for protein, although many pre-eclamptics will slip by unnoticed
  - excessive weight gain is a crude measure of fluid retention
  - thrombocytopaenia may be noted, although this is better used to track the severity of established disease
  - uric acid rises in pre-eclampsia. Again it is better used in tracking establishing disease
  - LFTs, creatinine clearance and coagulation screens including fibrin degradation products and more sensitively D-dimer levels. Disease requiring these investigations should be managed as an in-patient
  - the fetus must not be neglected as the circulatory changes of pre-eclampsia affect the placenta too. Growth retardation and hypoxia can occur

- ***action if screening is positive***: refer to an obstetrician. If proteinuric hypertension is found the patient should be admitted that day. The great mistake in dealing with pre-eclampsia is to underestimate it

---

Eclampsia

definition

A pre-eclamptic encephalopathy-induced convulsive disorder. It complicates <0.1% of all pregnancies in the UK.

presentation

Eclampsia may follow a period of time when pre-eclampsia was known. It may, on the other hand, be the first presentation of the disorder. It has been recorded as occurring as early as sixteen weeks into pregnancy and as late as twenty-three days after delivery. Half will present before labour. Over half of those presenting in the puerperium will do so more than forty-eight hours after delivery.

complications

Complications range from cerebrovasular damage including cortical blindness through the other endothelial damage syndromes (liver, kidney, coagulation system, placenta). The HELLP syndrome of haemolysis, elevated liver enzymes and low platelets is a particularly sinister combination.

treatment

In primary care, the first priority is to keep the mother safe (recovery position, airway attention etc) and to administer diazepam intravenously to abort the seizure. Immediate transfer to secondary care is required. Management may be shared between obstetricians and intensive care physicians.

Pre-term labour

Pre-term labour occurs before 37 weeks' gestation and accounts for 6–8% of deliveries (RCOG (i),1995). There is a strong link with genital tract infection and socio-behavioural markers for infection. All cases need to be referred to an obstetric unit urgently. Tocolysis is an option if labour is excessively pre-term but infection will need to be diligently sought in all cases. It is wise to examine the cervix aseptically (unless placenta praevia is suspected) to assess the imminence of delivery.

Premature rupture of membranes

Premature rupture of membranes is defined as rupture of the membranes before the onset of labour (at whatever gestation) and occurs in 4–18% of pregnancies, accounts for 50% of preterm deliveries and 10% of perinatal deaths, mainly from respiratory distress (RCOG (ii), 1995). It can be caused by trauma to the membranes but is usually the consequence of fragility of the membranes themselves. The membranes may be naturally weak or may have been weakened by infection. This may explain the link between bacterial vaginosis and pre-term delivery. The membranes can be subject to excessive pressure when the cervix has dilated leaving the forewaters unsupported. Infection is both a significant cause and complication of PROM. Diagnosis is made on observing liquor in the vaginal vault on 'sterile' speculum examination. If a sterile speculum is not available refer to an obstetrician for investigation even though many cases will prove to be urinary leakage. Maternal and fetal infection and pre-term delivery are the principal and significant complications. There is no place for management in the primary care setting; refer.

Puerperal affective disorder

Puerperal affective disorder blights many families. There are a range of presentations ranging from transient tearfulness to the frankly psychotic. In more severe cases there is a significant risk of suicide and infanticide. Puerperal psychiatric disorder can severely damage a marital relationship as well as impede the infant's development.

Presentations

the blues

This classically occurs on the fourth or fifth day after delivery. It may be preceded by a day or so of euphoria and elation. If mild and transient, support from the healthcare professional with encouragement and reassurance from the woman's family and friends may be all that is required.

postpartum depression

Postpartum depression has much in common with depressive disorder in the non pregnant state. A prior history of depressive disorder is not uncommon. Traumatic delivery including Caesarean section may be implicated. It usually presents within the first fortnight. Low mood, inappropriately poor sleep, lack of pleasure in motherhood, unworthy feelings, undue anxiety about the baby, restlessness and agitation are all signs to be alert for. Anti-depressants, either tricyclic or serotonin re-uptake inhibitors are commonly used. Progesterone has been suggested as a remedy but without good evidence of any effect. Oestrogens have been shown to be effective (as they are in premenstrual and peri-menopausal affective disorder). Oestrogens are administered in similar doses and formulations to those used in the menopause. Specialist psychiatric help should be obtained sooner rather than later. There is a strong case for management in dedicated mother and baby units. Compulsory admission to hospital under sections of the Mental Health Act may be required.

puerperal psychosis

This usually resembles manic depressive psychosis. Auditory and visual hallucinations are common features. A prior history is not uncommon. Lithium prophylaxis in subsequent pregnancies can be effective. Urgent specialist psychiatric involvement is vital. The suicide and infanticide risk is real.

thyroid disorder

Thyroid disorder is not uncommon in the puerperium and may present with a mood disorder. See the section below on 'Thyroid disorder'.

Treatment options

Sensitive proactive enquiry of maternal mood in the puerperium will unmask many cases of low grade depression. Many women attribute their malaise to the expected exhaustion of motherhood. Early intervention in the form of cognitive behavioural therapy or anti-depressant drugs can transform the situation. Untreated PND blights lives, damages relationships and can even compromise the social development of the child (Barclay C *et al*, 1998).

supportive care

Supportive care from family, friends and health professionals is vital and in mild and transient cases of mood disorder may be all that is required.

progesterone

Progesterone has been recommended by some people but without controlled trial evidence of benefit. Anecdotal reports of benefit exist. If a genuine clinical benefit is required then progesterone cannot be recommended; probably a relatively harmless placebo is preferable.

oestrogens

Oestrogens have been shown to produce improvement in hormone-related mood disorder in women (postpartum, peri-menopausal, premenstrual). Transdermal oestradiol 2x100 mcg patches twice weekly produced a significant improvement in one placebo-controlled trial (Gregoire *et al*, 1996).

antidepressants

Most tricyclics or SSRIs are thought to be safe in breast feeding mothers but see *Table 7.4* and consult *BNF* for data. Of the SSRIs, fluoxetine has the longest track record of safety for use in pregnancy and the puerperium. One recent study found its use in non-psychotic postnatal depression was as effective as six sessions of behavioural counselling. Giving counselling and fluoxetine therapy concurrently did not enhance improvement (Appleby L *et al*, 1997).

mother and baby units

These can transform life for affected families. Admission to a general psychiatric ward is a definite second best.

psychotherapy

Psychotherapy has a place at the secondary/tertiary level.

neuroleptics, lithium and ECT

These are the province of the specialist. If the situation is severe enough for these measures to be considered it is by definition outside the remit of the primary care professional.

Rhesus isoimmunization

The incidence of Rhesus isoimmunization and haemolytic disease of the new-born has dropped dramatically since the introduction of anti-D immunoglobulin immunization programmes in the early 1970s. The perinatal mortality rate, which had been running at around 120/100,000 live births, dropped to 1.5/100,000 by 1989. However, strict adherence to immunization protocols does not guarantee protection. In a large Scottish study, 53 of 71 mothers became sensitised despite the programme (Hughes, 1994). A significant number of cases still occur because anti-D is not given during threatened abortion or even after delivery. Lack of supplies and cost are the main argument against prophylactically immunizing Rh-D negative women at 28 weeks gestation. See *Table 6.9* for list of situations where anti-D immunoglobulin should be given. Other irregular antibodies have assumed importance as the incidence of Rhesus isoimmunization has dropped; these include anti-Kell and anti-Duffy antibodies.

Table 6.9: Situations where anti-D immunoglobulin should be given

Anti-D immunoglobulin should be given intramuscularly to all Rh-D negative women following:
stillbirth
amniocentesis
abortion/miscarriage
chorionic villus sampling
delivery of Rh-D positive infant
external cephalic version of breech
transfusion of Rh-D incompatible blood

Risk scoring in pregnancy

Risk scoring in pregnancy appears to have little to offer. Cases that are prospectively identifiable as being at higher than usual risk of adverse maternal or neonatal outcome are in the main quite obvious; for example, high order multiple pregnancy, the diabetic, the significantly hypertensive. If risk scoring is to act as a true screen (see 'Screening in gynaecology', ' General principles' in *Chapter 1*) and identify apparently healthy women and pregnancies that are 'at risk', then the conditions being screened for should be defined, and an acceptable test applied which is able to identify them with sensitivity and specificity. At present in the UK, there is no acceptable screen that can be offered to the asymptomatic which will predict, for example, pre-eclampsia and premature labour. The available risk score systems formally identify women already known to be candidates for consultant obstetrician care during pregnancy and delivery. In other words, they are check-lists and protocols. Perhaps the only true predictor of adverse outcome in the asymptomatic is socio-economic grouping as a risk factor for pre-term delivery. Screening tests have to be both acceptable to the target population and have precision. Questioning about social class would be unacceptable and lacks precision.

Rubella infection

Rubella infection is a potential disaster if acquired by the mother as a primary infection in the first trimester of pregnancy. The full congenital rubella syndrome includes hepatosplenomegaly, jaundice, cataract, cardiac defects, high tone deafness, microcephaly, microphthalmia and cerebral palsy. Infection is diagnosed by finding rubella specific IgM in the maternal blood. A history of German measles is too unreliable for diagnostic purposes. The incubation period is 14–21 days. IgM will be detectable for 8–12 weeks after the rash has cleared up. The earlier in pregnancy rubella is contracted the lower the transmission rate but the greater the risk of damage if fetal infection occurs (see *Table 6.10*). First trimester primary rubella is generally followed by termination of pregnancy.

Table 6.10: Rubella infection and transplacental transmission rates

gestation in weeks with rubella rash	congenital rubella infection rate
0–4	60%
4–8	25%
8–12	10%
12–16	5%

Rubella vaccination

Rubella vaccination is contraindicated in pregnancy and vaccinated women are advised to avoid pregnancy for 12 weeks. However, a study from the United States found that no increase in congenital anomaly was found in women who had been inadvertently vaccinated in pregnancy or who conceived quickly after vaccination (Preblud and Williams, 1985).

Seat belts in pregnancy

One of the listed causes of placental abruption is trauma. The commonest significant trauma in pregnancy is road traffic accident. The best advice to women in the later stages of pregnancy who wish to travel by car is to wear seat belts but to ensure that the belt does not cross the uterus. This can be achieved by ensuring that the lap part of a three point belt is placed low down crossing the suprapubic area between the iliac bones. The shoulder part of the belt should be placed to cross over above the uterus. Seat belts can cause abdominal trauma but their omission cannot be justified in pregnancy.

Skin changes caused by pregnancy

(See also skin conditions coinciding with pregnancy, *Chapter 7*). Skin changes in pregnancy can be divided neatly into physiological changes, particular dermatoses of pregnancy and the effect of pregnancy on established skin conditions. The latter is discussed in the next chapter. There is some overlap between the two.

Physiological skin changes in pregnancy

- **acne** may occur only in pregnancy. Sebaceous gland hyperplasia is common and produces the familiar Montgomery's tubercles of early pregnancy. Topical benzoic acid may be used. Low strength topical corticosteroids may help too. If severe acne develops in the presence of virilisation, androgen secreting tumour must be suspected

- **haemangiomata** can develop in pregnancy especially on the head and neck. Epulis (haemangioma of the gum) is described. They abate in the puerperium

- **hair** is rarely a problem. Hair loss after pregnancy is the norm and is caused by a hormonal telogen effluvium. It may resemble a male distribution. It relents by six months
- **milia** represents sebaceous hyperplasia
- **nails** may become brittle and fissured in pregnancy
- **oedema** affects half of all pregnancies. It is generally pedal. Pitting and generalised oedema should prompt screening for pre-eclampsia and renal disorder
- **pigmentation** is a universal feature in pregnancy affecting the face, breast, areola, linea alba (nigra) and anogenital areas. Freckles may darken. Melasma is not uncommon
- **pruritis** is extremely common affecting almost one in five pregnancies. Everyday causes must be considered (atopy, urticaria, scabies etc). A small number of cases will be presenting with a dermatosis of pregnancy. The rest will be experiencing pruritis as a manifestation of cholestasis of pregnancy etc (see 'Jaundice' above). This is the result of the effects of placental hormones on the liver. This presents in the last trimester and abates after delivery. A similar problem can complicate use of the combined oral contraceptive

pill. Calamine lotion may relieve, but more severe cases require anti-histamines. Rarely cholestyramine and even induction of labour may be indicated
- **purpura** can occur spontaneously, especially on the legs, perhaps due to raised hydrostatic pressure. Always investigate for more significant causes (platelet count, coagulation studies etc)
- **spider naevi** in the superior vena cava drainage areas are common in pregnancy. They usually regress after delivery. Consider hepatic disease
- **striae gravidarum** or stretch marks also occur in Cushing's disease and in obesity. There is a familial link. They are commoner in multiple pregnancy. Collagen quality reflecting lifelong nutrition may be involved. Emollients are often used but of unknown benefit
- **varicosities** due to increased hydrostatic pressure in the legs, compression of veins in the pelvis and haemorrhoidal areas and as a result of the relaxant properties of progesterone. All contribute to varicosities, particularly varicose veins in the legs, vulva and anal areas

---

Dermatoses of pregnancy

There are numerous skin conditions that may occur in pregnancy some of which have an auto-immune mechanism. The four conditions listed here are the only ones that will be seen with any frequency by the primary care professional. The involvement of a dermatologist is recommended for anything other than mild disorder.

pemphigoid gestationis (herpes gestationis)

This is a rare but important condition with vesicle formation on intense pruritic erythematous plaques. It can present at any time from the first trimester until the puerperium. Its differential diagnoses are polymorphic eruption of pregnancy and bullous pemphigoid.

The plaques develop peri-umbilically and spread radially. They may form wheals. It is more common in trophoblastic disease and there is a relation between it and paternal immunology. It is commoner in women with the same HLA group that is associated with Graves' disease, rheumatoid arthritis and juvenile onset diabetes mellitus. Exacerbations occur more severely in subsequent pregnancies with the same father. It can flare up if the combined oral contraceptive pill is used. Lactation appears to suppress it. Treatment should be under dermatological supervision and include anti-histamines, topical fluorinated steroids and prednisolone.

polymorphic eruption of pregnancy (PEP)

PEP is not uncommon (1:240 pregnancies) and presents with pruritis and urticaria in and around striae gravidarum. It is far commoner in primigravidas and in multiple gestation. Mild recurrence in subsequent pregnancy may occur. It presents well into the third trimester and is treated with anti-histamines and topical corticosteroids. Fetal DNA has been isolated from maternal lesions and may be the cause of the problem.

prurigo of pregnancy (*prurigo gestationis*)

This affects slightly fewer pregnancies than PEP and presents in the mid-trimester with a papular eruption which is pruritic. The rash affects the extensor surface of the limbs and the abdomen. The itch abates with delivery but the plaques may persist for some time afterwards. It may be linked with an atopic constitution. Treatment is with anti-histamines and topical coricosteroids.

pruritic folliculitis of pregnancy

Pruritic folliculitis of pregnancy is probably one end of the acneform spectrum. It is associated with follicular erythematous patches and may respond to topical benzoyl peroxide and topical corticosteroids.

Thromboembolic disorder

Thromboembolic disorder is covered above in the section on 'Postpartum collapse'. All causes of postpartum collapse can occur in pregnancy too.

Toxoplasmosis

Toxoplasmosis presents several dilemmas. The first relates to preconceptual and antenatal screening. The prerequisites for screening tests are presented in *Chapter 1*. The second relates to therapy which, although backed by animal experimentation data, has never been tested in a randomised way in humans despite widespread use in France and Belgium. Recent studies have however shown that spiramycin, pyrimethamine and folinic acid showed a good response. Toxoplasmosis produces a congenital infection most frequently when contracted late in pregnancy. Paradoxically, it is early pregnancy primary toxoplasmosis that produces the worst congenital disease. A recent study from Sheffield found one new case in over 1,600 pregnant women surveyed for at least 500 days each. The sero-positive prevalence rate was 9.9% and the only new case was known prior to the index pregnancy (Zadik, 1995). Repeated screening through pregnancy of the 90% seronegatives would have been a massive undertaking. Testing of any seroconverters would have to include consideration of cordocentesis, a procedure with a significant fetal mortality rate. The incidence of congenital toxoplasmosis in England and Wales is between ten and twenty cases per annum. The pragmatic approach is therefore to concentrate on avoidance of risk behaviour (listed in *Chapter 4*). If exposure is suspected serial antibody levels and management in conjunction with the local infectious disease specialist is advisable. There is no place for routine screening in the British obstetric population. Toxoplasmosis is a significant problem in the immunosuppressed.

Urinary incontinence

Antenatal urinary incontinence

There is unfortunately little to offer women with pregnancy-related urinary incontinence. Obviously urinary tract infection should be excluded and one must be clear the fluid leaking is indeed urine and not vaginal secretion or amniotic fluid. In the case of genuine stress incontinence which will have pre-dated the pregnancy, a well fitted polythene vaginal ring pessary can give excellent relief. With the anatomical changes of pregnancy a larger ring may be required. It may also be prudent in to take a swab for bacteriological analysis periodically. For the majority of women who leak during pregnancy, the reassurance that it almost always clears up after delivery may be of some comfort.

Postnatal urinary incontinence

Postnatal urinary incontinence is complained of by one in five women after normal delivery and is usually a new symptom. The incidence is lower if Caesarean section has been performed. The mechanism appears to be pelvic nerve damage caused by compression. As nerves repair, the problem usually resolves. Almost half of all women who have had three vaginal deliveries will have experienced urinary incontinence at some time. The bad news is that pelvic floor exercises do not appear to be helpful in reducing the incidence or shortening the duration of the problem. The important factor is pelvic nerve regeneration and that takes time. Prevention of nerve damage may be achieved if the duration of active pushing in the second stage is limited. The role of forceps delivery is unclear. They may, themselves, cause nerve compression but, on the other hand, they are generally reserved for use in cases where there has already been significant fruitless pushing and compression of the pelvic nerves.

Urinary tract infection

Urinary tract infection is a major complication in pregnancy. It is often masked by the pregnancy and so presents late. If suspected, it should be vigorously investigated and treated. Follow up urine cultures after treatment are advisable to ensure eradication has been achieved. Asymptomatic bacteriuria is present in 3–8% of pregnancies. It can lead to acute cystitis and pyelonephritis and renal scarring. A single asymptomatic screening urine culture will detect 80% of women with asymptomatic bacteriuria. A second screen will boost the pick-up rate to 95%. UTI may be linked to pre-term labour and delivery. It is common in higher socio-economic groups. Pyelonephritis, which may occur in as many as

30% of those with untreated asymptomatic bacteriuria, is characterised by fever, loin pain, cystitis and a positive urine culture. Recurrent infection may warrant prophylaxis. Urine culture should be performed in all pregnant women at booking. The older cephalosporins and nitrofurantoin are generally recommended (see *Chapter 7*, 'Anti-infection agents').

Varicella-zoster

Chickenpox can complicate pregnancy and the puerperium. It is estimated that one in ten adults have never had chickenpox and are therefore susceptible. Adult primary disease is generally more severe than in childhood and carries a 1:400 risk of pneumonitis and a 1:1000 risk of encephalitis. It appears that maternal shingles is not a cause of fetal/neonatal problems. Acyclovir has been used in pregnancy although it is unlicensed for such use. Zoster immune globulin has a place but, as with acyclovir, should be managed by a specialist in infectious diseases. Those wishing to know more could profitably read a short review by Venkatesan (1996) and RCOG Guidelines No 13.

- *congenital varicella syndrome* can occur when a primary infection occurs in a non-immune mother. The highest risk is between 13–20 weeks' gestation. Even during this time the full syndrome (hypoplastic limbs, dermal scarring, microcephaly, hydrocephally and eye problems) is uncommon

- *gestational chickenpox infection* should be managed in conjunction with an infectious diseases specialist and the obstetrician. Zoster immune globulin may be used. Acyclovir may have a place too. Not a primary care problem

- *gestational chickenpox exposure* in early pregnancy in women with no previous history of chickenpox should prompt chickenpox antibody assay on the same day. In an exposed non-immune mother, especially before twenty weeks' gestation, there may be a role for Zoster immune globulin. Although this may not prevent the maternal exanthem from appearing it will almost certainly protect the fetus. The incubation period from exposure to rash is around ten days

- *neonatal chickenpox* can be severe. In the baby of a non-immune mother, or where the mother sustains a primary infection within one week of delivery, the baby will have no passive immunity and Zoster immune globulin has a definite place. Consult a paediatrician or infectious diseases specialist urgently

- *maternal shingles* during pregnancy does not appear to carry a risk of congenital varicella syndrome to the fetus

Vitamin K

The 'koagulation factor' is involved in haemostasis. Deficiency leads to a haemorrhagic tendency. Lack of vitamin K causes haemorrhagic disease of the new-born which presents with spontaneous bleeding and, in the late onset variety, with intracranial haemorrhage. Children at especial risk of HDN include:

- the preterm
- the instrumentally delivered
- the asphyxiated
- breast fed babies
- babies born in the spring time
- babies with liver disease
- jaundiced babies (and babies of jaundiced mothers)
- maternal use of certain anticoagulants, NSAIDs and rifampicin.

Guidelines for the administration of Vitamin K are given in *Table 6.11*.

The *BNF* gives the following information on administering vitamin K:

- Phytomenadione (Konakion) 2 mg/ml. 0.5 ml ampoule

NB: Also available as 10 mg/ml ampoule which is **NOT FOR USE IN NEONATES**. (1mg=1,000 mcg)

Table 6.11: Guidelines for administration of Vitamin K to neonates

	British Paediatric Association Guidelines
1.	Vitamin K as Konakion in a dose of 500 mcg should be given orally to all babies at birth
2.	Vitamin K as Konakion in a dose of 100 mcg should be given by injection to infants at special risk where oral administration is not possible
3.	In fully breast fed babies, booster doses shuld be given at ten days and six weeks to avoid late haemorrhagic disease
4.	Infants fed on formula milk (which is supplemented with vitamin K) do not require additional doses
5.	Konakion is not licensed for oral administration but is used routinely as no other preparation is available. Local policies are common

Source: British Paediatric Association (1992) Report of Expert Committee, London

NB: These guidelines will probably be revised in the light of the two 1995 studies proving that intramuscular Vitamin K does not cause childhood leukaemia

Vitamin K and childhood cancer

Golding (1992) suggested that vitamin K administration was causally associated with the development of certain childhood cancers, especially leukaemia. At the time a leading paediatric authority stated in response that 'the risk of haemorrhagic disease is certain, that of cancer is not' and the paper was heavily criticised for methodological flaws. Two papers published in 1996 (von Kries R *et al* and Ansell P *et al)* have proved that vitamin K is not a cause of leukaemia and recommended that intramuscular prophylaxis be resumed.

Vomiting

Vomiting see 'Hyperemesis gravidarum', but always consider that other causes of this symptom/sign may be responsible.

Useful addresses

- SANDS: The Stillbirth and Neonatal Death Society, 28 Portland Place, London W1N 4DE
  Telephone 0171 436 5881
  (SANDS has a comprehensive network of support groups nationwide)

References

Ansell P *et al* (1996) Childhood leukaemia and intramuscular vitamin K: findings from a case-control study. *Br Med J* **313**: 204–5

Appleby L *et al* (1997) A controlled study of fluoxetine and cogitive behaviour counselling in the treatment of postnatal depression. *Br Med J* **314**: 932–6

Barclay C, Bazire S (1998) Depression before and after pregnancy. *Update* **57**: 622–625

CMO Communication (1992) *Management and Prevention of Listeriosis and other Food-borne Infections in Pregnancy*. PL/CMO (92)19

Drugs and Therapeutics Bulletin (1995) Routine iron supplements in pregnancy are unnecessary. *Drug Ther Bull* **32**: 30–1

Enkin M, Keirse M, Chalmers I (1994) *A Guide to Effective Care in Pregnancy and Childbirth*. Oxford University Press, Oxford

Frigo P *et al* (1998) Hyperemesis gravidarum associated with Helicobacter pylori seropositivity. *Obstet Gynecol* 91: 615–17

Golding J *et al* (1992) Intramuscular Vitamin K and pethidine given during labour. *Br Med J* **305**: 341–6

Gregoire AJP *et al* (1996) Transdermal oestrogen for treatment of severe postnatal depression. *Lancet* **347**: 930–3

Gupta S *et al* (1997) Women and HIV. B*r J Fam Plan* **23**: 83–7

Hughes RG *et al* (1994) Causes and clinical consequences of Rhesus (D) haemolytic disease of the new-born: a study of a Scottish population. *Br J Obstet Gynaecol* **101**: 297–300

Lucassen P *et al* (1998) Effectiveness of treatments for infantile colic: systematic review. *Br Med J* **316**: 1563–9

Preblud SR, Williams NM (1985) Fetal risk associated with rubella vaccination: implications for vaccinating susceptible women. *Obstet Gynecol* **66**: 121–3

RCOG (i) (1995) *Infection and Preterm Labour*. Divers M. PACE review 95/12 for the Royal College of Obstetricians and Gynaecologists, London

RCOG (ii) (1995) *Premature Rupture of the Membranes. Maternal and Perinatal Complications*. Cararach V. PACE review 95/08 for the Royal College of Obstetricians and Gynaecologists, London

SANDS (1991) *Miscarriage, Stillbirth and Neonatal Death. Guidelines for Professionals*. Available from SANDS, 28 Portland Place, London W1N 4DE. Telephone 0171 436 5881.

Stagno S *et al* (1986) Primary cytomegalovirus infection in pregnancy. *JAMA* **256** 1904–8

Steer P *et al* (1995) Relation between maternal haemoglobin concentration and birthweight in different ethnic groups. *Br Med J* **310**: 489–91

Venkatesan P (1996) Chickenpox in pregnancy: how dangerous? *Practitioner* **240**: 256–9

von Kries R *et al* (1996) Vitamin K and childhood cancer: a population based case-control study in Lower Saxony, Germany. *Br Med J* **313**: 199–203

Zadik PM *et al* (1995) Low incidence of primary infection with toxoplasma among women in Sheffield: a seroconversion study. *Br J Obstet Gynaecol* **102**: 608–10

Further reading

Bull MJV (1994) Review (on vitamin K and the neonate). *Diplomat* **1**: 70–4

CMO Communication (1992) *Prophylaxis against Vitamin K Deficiency Bleeding in Infants*. PL/CMO(92)20

Editorial (1994) Vitamin K. The controversy. *Br Med J* **308**: 867–8

Hull D (1992) Childhood cancer and vitamin K. *Br Med J* **305**:326–7

pregnancy and the puerperium (2) coincidental conditions

This chapter lists a variety of conditions and therapies that are either important or encountered with some frequency in women of childbearing age. I have tried to avoid overlap with the previous chapter by concentrating in this chapter on conditions and therapies incidental to pregnancy. In appropriate instances, data is presented in tabular form only.

The system used in this chapter for classifying the use of drugs in relation to pregnancy and the puerperium is that of the United States' Federal Drugs Agency. The FDA classification of teratogenesis is given in *Box 7.1* (opposite).

Chapter contents

Boxes and tables

Classification of drugs for use in pregnancy and the puerperium

Box 7.1: The FDA classification of drugs in relation to pregnancy

FDA classification of drugs	FDA advice
A	controlled studies in women have failed to show a risk in the first trimester and the risk of fetal harm seems remote
B	either animal tests do not show a risk but there have been no human studies, or animal studies show a risk but human studies have failed to show a risk to the fetus
C	either animal studies show teratogenic or embryocidal effects but there are no controlled studies in women, or there are no studies in either animals or humans
D	definite evidence of risk to the fetus exists but the benefits in certain circumstances (eg. life-threatening situations) may make use acceptable
X	fetal abnormalities have been shown in animals or humans or both, and the risk outweighs any possible benefits

Source: *Drugs in Pregnancy and Lactation,* Briggs *et al*
(The FDA classification covers drugs that are available [even if only illicitly] in the United States)

Alcohol (FDA: D)

Alcohol is a fetal teratogen. Chronic heavy alcohol ingestion is associated with the fetal alcohol syndrome (FAS). Unfortunately even moderate alcohol intake (circa 2 u/day) may be associated with fetal growth retardation. Even more worrying is the knowledge that this level of alcohol ingestion can have permanent effects on the pregnancy before the mother realises that she is pregnant. There is a very strong case, therefore, for stopping alcohol ingestion before conception and remaining alcohol-free throughout pregnancy (or at least until the second trimester when organogenesis is complete). Bingeing may be as harmful as chronic heavy drinking. Monitoring alcohol ingestion with serial MCV and GT estimations is masked by pregnancy-induced changes.

- **nutritional problems** are common among heavy drinkers. Trace element deficiencies may exist (zinc, copper) and there are commonly vitamin deficiency states (folate, thiamine, pyridoxine)
- **fetal alcohol syndrome** is seen in the offspring of heavy drinkers and alcoholics. The characteristic features are the facial anomalies of elongated philtrum, narrow palpebral

fissure, epicanthic folds associated with both growth and mental retardation. Although the facial dysmorphic features may regress with age, the mental retardation does not

- **breast feeding**: alcohol passes freely to the milk and concentrations equate with maternal blood levels. Regular heavy drinking by the mother may impede psychomotor development of the breast fed infant, although mental development is apparently unaffected. Heavy bingeing may lead to sedation of the infant

Analgesia

Table 7.1: Analgesics

Drug	FDA category	Notes
aspirin	C	risk factor rises to D in third trimester. May compromise clotting in neonate. Association with APH, prolonged pregnancy and labour. Low dose aspirin regimes appear safe(er). Very low transfer to milk
paracetamol	B	crosses placenta, can cause liver damage in maternal overdose. N-acetylcystein is not considered teratogenic. Low level transfer to milk
codeine	C	respiratory depression in labour, withdrawal symptoms after birth. Codeine may be present in cough remedies
NSAIDs		see 'Anti-inflammatories' below
pentazocine	B	no data on breast feeding
diamorphine	B	NB: illicit heroin may be adulterated. Respiratory depression of neonate. Fetal abstinence syndrome in regular (ab)users. Breast milk levels in habitual users can induce neonatal addiction
naloxone	B	no data on breast feeding. Severe reaction in narcotic habituated neonates reported

Sources: *BNF* and *Drugs in Pregnancy and Lactation*, Briggs *et al*

Anticoagulation

Women using anticoagulants before pregnancy should attend a specialist pre-pregnancy clinic. Heparin is probably the drug of choice. Warfarin, which must be avoided in the first trimester, can cause anomaly at any time in pregnancy. See *Table 7.2*.

Table 7.2: Anticoagulants

Drug	FDA category	Notes
heparin	C	does not cross placenta or enter breast milk. Not known to be teratogenic. Dose-related osteopaenia in mother
warfarin	D	risk factor X according to manufacturers. Embryopathic fetal warfarin syndrome if used 6–9 weeks' gestation, CNS damage at any stage in pregnancy. Warfarin appears safe in breast feeding

Sources: *BNF* and *Drugs in Pregnancy and Lactation*, Briggs *et al*

Always check the appropriate literature before prescribing anything in pregnancy and the puerperium. The responsibility for prescribing resides with the prescriber. The above data provides general guidelines only

Anticonvulsants

See *Table 7.3*. Their use presents dilemmas in pregnancy. Many anticonvulsants are teratogens. There has to be a balance between the maternal interest and the avoidance of fetal damage. This is an area of particular importance in preconceptual advice and, just as diabetic girls should be acquainted with the risks to their babies of unplanned pregnancies, so too should girls and women taking anticonvulsant medication. If pregnancy is desired, the active involvement of an obstetrician and/or neurologist with a particular interest is vital.

- **Pregnancy can affect epilepsy**: an increase in seizure frequency may be seen especially in women who were already experiencing one or more seizures per month. Seizure frequency may be increased in later pregnancy as sleep disturbance increases. The risk of seizure in labour is quoted at 1% and is frequently attributed to hyperventilation
- **Epilepsy can affect pregnancy**: although the hypoxic insult to the fetus of maternal convulsion is usually well tolerated, status epilepticus is associated with a significant fetal mortality. The drugs used in pregnancy may have teratogenic effects, particularly neural tube and cardiac defects and oro-facial clefts (epileptic women have a higher incidence of oro-facial clefts in their relatives anyway). Multiple drug therapy increases the teratogenic risk. Some anti-convulsants interfere with vitamin K metabolism and can predispose to haemorrhagic disease of the new-born. Vitamin K at delivery is advisable (See *Chapter 6*)

General advice includes:

- avoidance of unplanned pregnancy by prescribing a higher dose contraceptive pill (see *Chapter 3*)
- education of girls and young women on preconceptual preparation
- mono-therapy if possible
- folate supplements at high dose before conception (especially important)
- CSM advises pre-pregnancy counselling on fetal abnormality
- screen pregnancies carefully for NTD and other anomalies
- Vitamin K supplement before delivery to mother and after delivery to baby.

Table 7.3: Anticonvulsants

Drug	FDA classification	Fetal/neonatal effects
carbamazepine	C	NTD, folate depletion, vitamin K depletion. Lactation use considered safe
chlormethiazole	–	depressed neonatal respiration. For eclampsia only. Lactation use considered safe
clonazepam	C	see diazepam
diazepam	D	hypotonia, respiratory depression, withdrawal reaction. Lactation sedation
ethosuximide	C	teratogenic? No clear data. Considered safe in lactation
gabapentin	–	teratogenic. No data on lactation
lamotrigine	–	teratogenic. No data on lactation
methylbarbitone	–	see phenobarbitone
paraldehyde	–	only use in eclampsia. No data on lactation
phenobarbitone	D	digital and facial anomalies, folate depletion. Vitamin K depletion, long term learning difficulties. Passes to milk, mothers advised to watch for signs of sedation in infant
primidone	–	metabolises to phenobarbitone. Avoid in lactation
phenytoin	D	dysmorphic features, folate and vitamin K depletion. Possible transplacental carcinogen. Considered safe in breast feeding *
valproate	D	multisystem fetal anomalies reported including facial, cardiac and neural tube defects, folate depletion, neonatal bleeding and hepatotoxicity
vigabatrin	–	toxicity in animal studies (palate cleft in rabbit studies). No data on lactation *

Sources: *BNF* and *Drugs in Pregnancy and Lactation*, Briggs *et al*

Note:
* manufacturer advises avoid

Always check the appropriate literature before prescribing anything inpregnancy and the puerperium. The responsibility for prescribing resides with the prescriber. The above data provides general guidelines only

Antidepressants

Table 7.4: Antidepressants

Drug	FDA classification	Notes
tricyclics		
amitriptyline	D	teratogenic, not known to be harmful in lactation but use with caution
amoxapine	C	effects in pregnancy not known; avoid in lactation
clomipramine	D	no evidence of harm; withdrawal syndrome may occur in neonate. Cautious use in breast feeding; probably best avoided
desipramine	C	neonatal withdrawal syndrome; probably best avoided in lactation
dothiepin	D	no data available for use in pregnancy; probably best avoided in lactation
doxepin	C	some concerns on use in pregnancy; probably best avoided in lactation as may accumulate in baby and sedate
imipramine	D	possible association with cardiac defects; withdrawal syndrome may occur in neonate. Cautious use in breast feeding; probably best avoided
lofepramine	–	no data
maprotiline	B	not known to be harmful in pregnancy or lactation; cautious use
mianserin	–	no data
nortriptyline	D	teratogenic; not known to be harmful in lactation but use with caution
protriptyline	C	no data
trimipramine	–	no data
trazodone	C	little data; no teratogenic effects known; best avoided in lactation
viloxazine	–	no data
SSRIs		
citalopram	–	manufacturers advise use only if potential benefits outweigh unstated risks
fluvoxamine	–	manufacturers advise use only if potential benefits outweigh unstated risks
fluoxetine	B	no evidence of harm in pregnancy; no data on harm
nefazodone	–	manufacturers advise use only if potential benefits outweigh unstated risks
paroxetine	–	manufacturers advise use only if potential benefits outweigh unstated risks
sertraline	B	no evidence of harm in pregnancy; no data on harm. Adverse effects in animals. Probably best avoided in lactation
venlafaxine	–	manufacturers advise use only if potential benefits outweigh unstated risks
MAOIs		
isocarboxazid	C	increased risk of fetal malformation? Lactation: no data available
phenelzine	C	increased risk of fetal malformation? Lactation: no data available
tranylcypromine	C	increased risk of fetal malformation? Lactation: no data available
moclobemide	–	manufacturers advise avoid in pregnancy and lactation
Others		
Flupenthixol	–	extrapyramidal effects in neonate have been reported
tryptophan	–	contraindicated in pregnancy and lactation, an amino-acid. Hospital use only

Sources: *BNF* and *Drugs in Pregnancy and Lactation*, Briggs et al

Always check the appropriate literature before prescribing anything in pregnancy and the puerperium. The responsibility for prescribing resides with the prescriber. The above data provides general guidelines only

Anti-infection agents

Virus

There are few indications for the use of anti-viral agents in pregnancy, and even fewer in the primary care setting.

Table 7.5: Antiviral drugs

Drug	Route	FDA classification	Notes
acyclovir	oral/parenteral eye ointment skin cream	C	probably safe; no problem in lactation no data no data
amantadine	oral	C	few data; best avoided in lactation
famcyclovir	oral	–	*BNF* states 'see acyclovir'
podophyllin	topical	–	*BNF* states avoid. Teratogenic and neonatal death reported
zidovudine	oral	C	HIV use. No data on harm in pregnancy
ganciclovir	oral/parenteral	–	CMV use

Sources: *BNF* and *Drugs in Pregnancy and Lactation*, Briggs *et al*

Always check the appropriate literature before prescribing anything in pregnancy and the puerperium. The responsibility for prescribing resides with the prescriber. The above data provides general guidelines only

Bacterial infection

Table 7.6: Antibacterial drugs

Drug	Pregnancy	Breast feeding	Notes
aminoglycosides	x	caution	avoid if possible. Risk greatest with strepto-mycin. Topical gentamycin: use with caution
cephalosporins	caution	caution	not known to be harmful
chloramphenicol	x systemic caution topical	x systemic caution topical	safety of topical preparations not established. 'Grey syndrome': a theoretical risk
clavulanic acid	caution	√	
clindamycin	caution	caution	
clioquinol (topical)	caution	caution	no data on toxicity
fosformycin	caution	caution	not known to be harmful, but avoid if possible
fusidic acid	x systemic caution	x systemic caution	no data on topical cream formulation
macrolides	caution	caution	erythromycin not known to be harmful
metronidazole/tinidazole	caution	caution	toxicity in animal studies; avoid tinidazol in first trimester. Avoid single large doses in lactation
naladixic acid	caution	caution	few data; avoid in first trimester
nitrofurantoin	caution	?	do not use in pregnancy at term
penicillin	√	√	
other β lactam antibiotics	caution	caution	aztreonam is contraindicated in pregnancy and lactation
polymyxin	x	x	

Table 7.6: Antibacterial drugs (contd)

Drug	Pregnancy	Breast feeding	Notes
4-quinolones	caution	caution	arthropathy in animal studies
rifampicin	caution	caution	toxicity in high dose animal studies; risk of neonatal bleeding. Vitamin K needed. Drug passes into milk
sulphonomides	x	caution	third trimester fetal haemolysis and kernicterus risk especially in G6PD-deficient infants
tetracycline	x	x	
trimethoprim	caution	caution	a folate antagonist; theoretical first trimester teratogen

Sources: *BNF* and *Drugs in Pregnancy and Lactation*, Briggs et al

Notes:

✓   probably safe

x   contraindicated

Always check the appropriate literature before prescribing anything in pregnancy and the puerperium. The responsibility for prescribing resides with the prescriber. The above data provides general guidelines only

Fungi

Table 7.7: Antifungal drugs

Drug	Route	Pregnancy	Breast feeding	Notes
amphoteracin	oral/iv	caution	no data	
nystatin	oral, pr, pv, topical	poor effect	no data	
imidazoles eg. clotrimazole, miconazole	pv, topical	√	√	see data sheets for non-topical use
triazoles eg. fluconazole, itraconazole	oral	x	avoid	
griseofulvin	oral	x	caution	men should not try to produce pregnancy for 6 months after treatment has finished
terbinafine	oral, topical	caution	caution	

Note:

See also 'Candidiasis' in *Chapter 1*

Helminths, worms, protozoa

Treatment of most infestations can be deferred until after delivery to avoid exposure of the fetus to potential toxins. For example, the management of hookworm infestation is, unless the parasitic load is overwhelming, to supplement with iron and folic acid until delivery. However, four organisms exist which may be encountered in general practice and which demand treatment during pregnancy to reduce maternal morbidity and mortality. These are *entamoeba histolytica, malaria, giardia lamblia* and *ascariasis*. The last of these is probably the most commonly seen in this country although the request for anti-malarial chemoprophylaxis is increasing with the escalating popularity of long haul air travel vacations.

- ***Ascariasis lumbricoides*** or roundworm may be treated with pyrantel in pregnancy. The life cycle of the worm involves migration into the lung via the trachea. Obstetric deaths as a result have been reported. It is always worth seeking specialist help in these instances. The advice of an infectious disease specialist, the local drug information pharmacist and perhaps the obstetrician is advisable

- ***Malaria*** is usually easy to diagnose, but only if the diagnosis is suspected in the first place. The malarial parasites have a predilection for the placenta and in concert with the altered immune state of pregnancy can cause severe and even fatal disease. Pregnant women contemplating travel to endemic areas should seriously consider their motivations for taking such a risk (ie. do not go if at all possible). The risk of malaria is reduced by adequate chemoprophylaxis, but this carries with it its own burden of anxieties regarding its potential teratogenicity. Suspected cases need urgent investigation; indeed emergency admission to resolve the question and if necessary to avoid delay in instituting treatment. Prophylactic regimes require detailed and up to the minute data on drug resistance for safe prescribing. The data below can help in decision-making. If the traveller is pregnant and must travel to an endemic area discussion with a tropical medicine specialist is strongly recommended. The physical measures for avoiding bites should be emphasised. Insect repellents which have diethyltoluamide (DEET) in their formulation should not be used during pregnancy. Mosiguard which contains lemon and eucalyptus extracts is recommended instead (see *Table 7.8*).

- ***Entamoeba and giardia*** infestation in pregnancy need the involvement of an infectious diseases specialist

- ***Other protozoal infections*** mentioned in the *BNF* include trichomonas, which requires GUMed investigation and treatment; leishmaniasis, toxoplasmosis and pneumocystis, which require specialist involvement

- ***Other helminth infestations*** mentioned in the *BNF* include threadworms, tapeworms, hookworm, schistosomiasis, filariasis, guinea worm and strogyloides

Table 7.8: Antimalarial drugs

Drug	Pregnancy	Breast feeding	Comment
chloroquine	caution	√	
halofantrine	x	x	
mefloquine	x	x	avoid pregnancy for 3 months after use
primaquine	caution	caution	
proguanil	√	√	folate supplements essential
pyrimethamine	caution	caution	folate supplements essential
Fansidar®	–	–	no longer recommended for prophylaxis
Maloprim®	caution	caution	
quinine	x	√	
tetracycline	x	x	

Sources: *BNF, ABPI Data Sheet Compendium*

Notes:
√   probably safe
x   contraindicated

Always check the appropriate literature before prescribing anything in pregnancy and the puerperium. The responsibility for prescribing resides with the prescriber. The above data provides general guidelines only

Anti-inflammatories (NSAIDs)

Anti-inflammatories (NSAIDs) are widely available but should be used, if at all, with great caution in late pregnancy. The two potential effects are inhibition of labour (NSAIDs have been used as tocolytics) and via their effects on prostaglandin synthetase premature closure of the ductus arteriosus. The FDA classification of ibuprofen, indomethacin and naproxen is 'B' in the first two trimesters, but 'D' in the third trimester. NSAIDs appear to be safe in lactation. Briggs' *Drugs in Pregnancy and Lactation* found far more problems associated with indomethacin than ibuprofen. Briggs does not list many drugs which are popular in the UK (eg. diclofenac sodium).

Antipsychotics

See *Table 7.9*. In general terms it is better to use behavioural and psychotherapeutic treatments during pregnancy or if pregnancy is desired. Psychotropic drugs are listed very generally here. Anticonvulsant and antidepressant drugs are listed and tabulated above. In specific cases, discussion with a drug information pharmacist, psychiatrist and obstetrician interested in preconceptual care is advisable.

Table 7.9: Psychotropic drugs

Drug group	Lower risk	Moderate risk	Higher risk	Notes
neuroleptics	flupenthixol sulpiride	buterophenones, clozapine, lozapine, phenothiazines, risperidone	prochlorperazine	
anxiolytics and hypnotics	zopiclone	beta-blockers, buspirone, chloral, chlormethiazole, promethazine	benzodiazepines, zolpidem	
lithium	–	–	lithium	goitre and hypothyroidism; Ebstein's cardiac anomaly (rare)
others	–	anticholinergics, disulfiram, methadone, paraldehyde	diethylpropion, methadone	

Source: Bazire S (1998) *GP Psychotropic Handbook*. Quay Books

Always check the appropriate literature before prescribing anything in pregnancy and the puerperium. The responsibility for prescribing resides with the prescriber. The above data provides general guidelines only

Asthma

The consensus view is in favour of maintaining or achieving excellent asthma control in pregnancy. Rather than withdrawing prophylactic and therapeutic medications, asthmatic women should be women should be encouraged to continue with them. Best treatment involves inhaled medication which poses even less theoretical risk than oral preparaions. Uncontrolled asthma poses far greater risks to the fetus than the mother's medication.

Table 7.10: Drugs used in asthma

Drug	FDA classification	Notes
β mimetics		
salbutamol	–	*BNF* advises use with caution but does not state what to be cautious about!
terbutaline	B	as per salbutamol
bambutrol	–	manufacturer advises avoid in pregnancy
eformoterol	–	manufacturer advises avoid in pregnancy and lactation
fenoterol	B	as per salbutamol
reproterol	–	as per salbutamol
salmetrol	–	as per salbutamol
tulobuterol	–	manufacturer advises avoid in pregnancy
other adrenoreceptor stimulants		
adrenaline	C	only indicated in life threatening asthma
ephedrine and isoprenaline	C	*BNF* advises avoid if possible in any situation
orciprenaline	–	*BNF* advises avoid if possible in any situation
pseudoephedrine		*BNF* advises avoid if possible in any situation
antimuscarinics		
ipratropium/oxitropium	–	*BNF* advises caution in pregnancy
theophylline		
theophylline	–	can cause neonatal irritability, m/r preparations probably all right in lactation
aminophylline	–	as per theophylline
choline theophyllinate	–	as per theophylline
corticosteroids		
prednisolone (oral)	B	only used in severe asthma
beclomethasone	–	indicated for asthma in pregnancy and lactation
budesonide	–	as per beclomethasone
fluticasone	–	as per beclomethasone
chromoglycate		
sodium chromoglycate	–	as indicated for asthma in pregnancy and lactation
nedocromil	–	as per chromoglycate
leukotriene receptor antagonists		
montelukast	–	manufacturer advises avoid unless essential
zafirlukast	–	manufacturer advises use only if potential benefit outweighs risk. Present in breast milk, avoid in lactation

Principal sources: *MIMS*, November 1999; *BNF* **38**, September 1999

Always check the appropriate literature before prescribing anything in pregnancy and the puerperium. The responsibility for prescribing resides with the prescriber. The above data provides general guidelines only

Caffeine

Caffeine is one of the most common non-prescribed drugs taken world-wide. It is present in teas (including many herbal infusions), coffee, cola drinks as well as being a constituent of several popular combination analgesics and treatments for migraine. Heavy intake is associated with reduced fecundity and probably spontaneous abortion. Evidence of fetal toxicity is difficult to prove because simple analgesic use, tobacco smoking and alcohol consumption are all closely linked with caffeine consumption. Moderate intake probably has no adverse effects in pregnancy. The FDA classifies caffeine in group 'B'. Very high intake by nursing mothers can lead to irritability in the neonate whose excretion half life for caffeine is 80 hours.

Diabetes mellitus

Diabetes mellitus needs careful management beginning preconceptually and continuing through to the puerperium. The active involvement of a diabetologist and obstetrician is vital. Patient education on the importance of preparation for pregnancy must begin in the early teenage years. The principles are:

- **education** as mentioned above is vital. First presentation in a planned pregnancy in a diabetic who is truly unaware of preconceptual requirements suggests omission on the part of her attendants
- **insulin therapy** rather than oral hypoglycaemic agents is recommended. The detail of doses and schedules should be attended to by a diabetologist
- **euglycaemia** not only in pregnancy but preconceptually is vital if the incidence of major fetal anomaly is to equate with non-diabetic women
- **screening** for end organ damage is part of the preconceptual workup. Retinal state and renal function need assessment.

See also 'Altered glucose tolerance in pregnancy' *Chapter 6* and 'Preconceptual care' *Chapter 4*.

Hypertension

See *Table 7.11*. Presents either as chronic hypertension which pre-dates the pregnancy or as part of the pre-eclamptic process. It is possible for pre-eclampsia to be superimposed upon chronic hypertension. The principles of management of chronic hypertension are:

- **treat the mother rather than the pregnancy**: with the exception of severe accelerated hypertension the fetal interests are unaffected by maternal blood pressure. Pre-eclampsia is different; it causes endothelial damage that results in both fetal morbidity and the rise in maternal blood pressure. Renal function is of considerable prognostic importance in pregnancy

- **avoid all medication in the first trimester if possible**: if the maternal blood pressure is not too high and poses no immediate danger to the mother, it is permissible to stop antihypertensive medication. It may not be required again until the third trimester
- **be alert to the natural drop in blood pressure in the second trimester** of pregnancy. This may allow a delay in starting or restarting antihypertensive medication
- **be alert to the natural rise in blood pressure in the third trimester**: this will need to be sought diligently. Pre-eclampsia is more common in the chronic hypertensive
- **chronic hypertension and pre-eclampsia are linked**: women with chronic hypertension are at greater risk of developing pre-eclampsia. It may be useful to screen hypertensive women with serial urate and platelet counts through the second half of pregnancy. The former rise and the latter fall in pre-eclampsia
- **consider the cause of chronic hypertension**: the majority will have 'essential' hypertension. Some will have it as a result of renal disease. The remainder are rarities and result from phaeochromocytoma, Cushing's syndrome, Conn's syndrome, aortic coarctation.

Table 7.11: Anti-hypertensive drugs

Drug	Notes
β blockers	may cause IUGR, fetal bradycardia and hypoglycaemia. Short term use in third trimester only
diuretics	disadvantages in PET; mainly for heart failure
ACE inhibitors	teratogenic, fetal nephrotoxicity
calcium channel blockers	may interfere with initiation of labour
clonidine	not for primary care
prazocine	not for primary care
methyldopa	the drug with the longest and safest profile for use in pregnancy

|Illicit drug use

See *Table 7.12*. Use is far more common in the United States where cocaine use complicates up to one quarter of pregnancies in some urban areas. In this country tobacco and alcohol are the most common adverse drugs used in pregnancy and because of the scale of the problem they are discussed separately. Illicit drug use is less common, but more covert. Hard drug use requires money and is not infrequently linked with crime, prostitution and poor social circumstance. Because of needle sharing and sexual exposure, hepatitis B and HIV are more common in the illicit drug user.

In needle sharers there is a risk of Rhesus antibody formation in Rhesus D negative women. Drug abuse results in high risk of adverse outcome in pregnancy and should be managed in close concert with obstetricians, substance abuse specialists, mental health services and, where appropriate, the social services.

- **neonatal abstinence syndrome** is common in babies born to opiate drug abusing mothers. Irritability, a high pitched cry, nasal snuffles associated with gastro-intestinal disturbance and respiratory distress are typical. Coma and convulsion are possible. Severe NAS can be induced with rapidity in withdrawing neonates exposed to naloxone. Symptoms present within a few hours of birth in the babies of heroin addicts and in a day or so in babies of methadone using mothers.

Table 7.12: Illicit drugs

Drug	Notes
amphetamines	IUGR
alcohol	fetal alcohol syndrome; alcohol in breast milk; IUGR. Associations with trace element depletion
benzodiazepines	short term use of little worry. Floppy baby, depressed respiration in neonate, addictive, ?teratogenic
cocaine	teratogenic, IUGR, impairs psychomotor development, significantly higher APH in pregnancy, prematurity
crack cocaine	free base cocaine
'ecstasy'*	an amphetamine derivative
heroin	*in utero* withdrawal reactions, NAS shortly after birth, increases SIDS
LSD	teratogenic, phocomelia and amniotic band anomalies
marijuana	IUGR, ?chromosome damage
methadone	similar to heroin but longer half life reduces *in utero* withdrawal and delays NAS
narcotic antagonists	eg. pentazocin and naloxone. Can be particularly dangerous in the withdrawing neonate
solvents	maternal renal tubular acidosis, IUGR
tobacco	IUGR

Notes:
*   methylenedioxymethamphetamine (MDMA)
APH   ante-partum haemorrhage
IUGR   intrauterine growth retardation
NAS   neonatal abstinence syndrome
SIDS   sudden infant death syndrome

Inflammatory bowel disease

Inflammatory bowel disease is not uncommon in young women and therefore not uncommon in pregnancy even though there is a link between active disease and involuntary infertility. Poor pregnancy outcome appears to be associated with the first occurrence of disease in pregnancy and active or extensive disease present at the beginning of pregnancy. Ulcerative colitis has a tendency to relapse in the first trimester. Crohn's disease has a tendency to relapse in the puerperium. Women with colonic disease fare less well than those with isolated small bowel involvement. Treatment with prednisolone and sulphasalazine appears to be safe (although it is linked with reversible infertility in men). Azathioprine and methotrexate are not safe in pregnancy. Lomotil is advised against in pregnancy. Attention needs to be paid to nutritional factors and the advice of a gastroenterologist should be sought. Iron, folic acid, vitamin D as well as trace elements need to be considered. In both conditions, pregnancy is best deferred until the disease is quiescent and when medication is at a minimum.

Irritable bowel syndrome

Irritable bowel syndrome is a condition which is usually a diagnosis of exclusion and where treatment is empirical. During pregnancy antispasmodics and antidiarrhoeal preparations are contraindicated. After exclusion of alternative diagnoses (malignancy, inflammatory bowel disorder, hypothyroidism etc) treatment is aimed at providing sufficient fluid and fibre on which the bowel can work.

Migraine

Migraine is common but tends to be associated with hormonal withdrawal rather than the hormonal abundance of pregnancy. Thus, classical migraine tends to ease or abate in pregnancy. Occasionally however, migraine can present for the first time in pregnancy. Treatment is three pronged:

- *analgesics* should be simple, as discussed above. The occasional addition of an anti-emetic (eg. metoclopramide) is acceptable if the indication is compelling
- *prophylactic medication* consists of beta-blockers, such as propranolol to reduce the frequency of attacks and low dose aspirin to counteract the thrombotic potential during the vasospastic first phase of a migraine attack. The other usual prophylactics include pizotifen, which may be safe in pregnancy but the manufacturers advise avoidance and tricyclics which are not advisable in pregnancy
- *avoidance of contraindicated drugs in pregnancy*: these include all ergot derivatives and isometheptene mucate (Midrid). Sumatriptan is advised only with caution in pregnancy by its manufacturers.

Skin conditions coinciding with pregnancy

(See also skin conditions caused by pregnancy, *Chapter 6*). Skin conditions are common in women in their fertile years and, not surprisingly, commonly coincide with pregnancy. Five common dermatological conditions are considered here.

Acne vulgaris

The effects of pregnancy on acne are unpredictable. It may improve or indeed it may present in pregnancy for the first time.

- **Safe treatments** include topical benzoic acid, topical low potency corticosteroids. Erythromycin is not known to be harmful
- **Unsafe treatments** include tetracyclines, oral and systemic vitamin A derivatives, topical azelic acid

Condylomata accuminata

The fleshy viral warts that occur on the vulva and peri-anal areas are likely to grow in pregnancy. They may occasionally become so florid that vaginal delivery is precluded. There is a link between vulvovaginal condylomata and neonatal laryngeal warts.

- **Safe treatments** include cryocautery and diathermy
- **Unsafe treatments** include podophyllin application

Eczema

Eczema may improve or deteriorate in pregnancy. There is a link between atopy and prurigo of pregnancy. Eczema is more likely to deteriorate if pruritis develops in pregnancy.

- **Safe treatments** include emollients, low potency topical corticosteroids
- **Unsafe treatments** include possibly EPO (manufacturers advise caution)

Melanoma

Pregnancy is a condition accompanied by skin pigment changes. There is debate on the effect pregnancy has on the natural history of malignant melanoma. There are suggestions that new naevii developing in pregnancy or in the first year after delivery are marginally more likely to be malignant than at other times in life. The advice to the generalist regarding pigmented skin lesions is to be as vigilant and as cautious with pregnant and puerperal women, as with anyone else.

Psoriasis

The course of psoriasis is variable in pregnancy. An uncommon but serious variant of psoriasis may occur in pregnancy. Intertrigo herpetiformis is a pustular rash that occurs in skin flexures especially the inguinal area. It produces sterile pustules and can deteriorate into a systemic illness. It is linked with adverse fetal/neonatal outcome and should be managed by dermatologists and obstetricians.

- **Safe treatments** of psoriasis include emollients, low potency topical corticosteroids, tar preparations and dithranol
- **Unsafe treatments** include calcipitriol (Dovanex), cyclosporin, methotrexate, azathioprine and PUVA

Thyroid disease

See *Table 7.13*. Thyroid disease is common in women in the childbearing years but is under-represented in pregnancy because both hyperthyroidism and hypothyroidism reduce fertility. World-wide, iodine deficient endemic goitre is a major cause of maternal illness, pregnancy wastage and morbidity in the children of affected pregnancies. In this country goitre is usually sporadic, perhaps occurring due to iodine deficiency or sometimes caused by goitrogens. Some goitrogens can cause fetal goitre. Most will not cause problems unless there is associated iodine deficiency. Thyroid dysfunction in pregnancy is not uncommon. Thyroid dysfunction after delivery is common and under-recognised.

Table 7.13: Common potential goitrogens

Drug group	Drug examples
antithyroid drugs	carbimazole, propylthiouracil
iodine containing drugs	iodides, amiodarone, idoxuridine ophthalmic solution
other goitrogens	sulphonamides, sulphonylureas, acetazolamide, lithium, antihistamines, methylxanthines
foods	cabbage, cauliflower, sprouts, turnips, cassava, maize, calcium, fluoride, nitrates, sulphurated hydrocarbons found in certain drinking water

Sporadic goitre

Sporadic goitre may be the result of the thyrotropic effect of placental hormones (hCG). It is more common in hyperemetic women and in cases of trophoblastic disease. It may also be seen in iodine deficiency or goitrogens.

Hypothyroidism

Hypothyroidism complicates around nine per thousand pregnancies. Features include fatigue, hair loss and hair dryness, excessive weight gain, cold intolerance (unusual in pregnancy), muscle stiffness and carpal tunnel syndrome. It is associated with higher miscarriage and stillbirth rates. There is a higher incidence of ante and postpartum haemorrhage. During the first trimester the fetus is entirely dependent on maternal thyroid hormone and deficiency risks neuro-cretinism. Pre-eclampsia is more common, and indeed hypertension, proteinuria and oedema can be features of hypothyroidism too. Investigation of thyroid function is complicated by the physiological effects of pregnancy and blood samples should be accompanied by clear labelling of the presence and duration of gestation. Early involvement of an endocrinologist is recommended. Frequent monitoring through pregnancy and the puerperium is required. Thyroxin is the treatment.

Thyrotoxicosis

Thyrotoxicosis is less common than underactivity of the thyroid complicating just two per thousand pregnancies. Almost all will be due to Grave's disease. Three-quarters of cases will have been present before pregnancy. Those cases that do develop in pregnancy generally present at 10–15 weeks' gestation. The symptoms and signs include poor weight gain, ocular signs and tachycardia. A positive family history is common. In untreated cases, one quarter of babies will be stillborn, more than a half will be born pre-term and one fifth of mothers will develop a thyrotoxic crisis with a 10% maternal mortality rate. Pre-pregnancy preparation under the care of an endocrinologist is advisable for women with pre-existing disease who desire pregnancy. This will enable surgery and radio-iodine therapy to be considered and drug treatment optimised. Treatments include:

- *carbimazole* crosses the placenta and may cause fetal hypothyroidism. Disputed link with the anomaly aplasia cutis. Be alert for the rare but sinister agranulocytosis which is associated with its use
- *propylthiouracil* is the other main anti-thyroid drug. It is marginally preferable in pregnancy and in women who breast feed. However, women stabilised on carbimazole are not advised to change over

- β-**blockers** can be used symptomatically if strongly indicated while awaiting a response to anti-thyroid medication. There is an association between their use and poor fetal growth, fetal distress and hypoglycaemia
- **surgery** may very occasionally be indicated in pregnancy
- **radio-iodine** is contraindicated in pregnancy and in women breast feeding their infants. The fetal/neonatal thyroid takes up iodine with especial avidity.

Fetal/neonatal thyroid dysfunction

Thyroid problems in the fetus usually reflect the maternal condition and are the consequence of drugs given to the mother. Thyroid stimulating antibodies can cross the placenta and cause intrauterine thyrotoxicosis. This may be suspected if finding poor fetal growth and a persistent tachycardia (>160/min). Anti-thyroid drugs cross the placenta too and can induce fetal hypothyroidism and goitre. Radio-iodine, as already mentioned, is absolutely contraindicated. 'Block and replace' therapy is no longer recommended in pregnancy. Some authorities wean down anti-thyroid drugs in the third trimester in the fetal interests, but there is a risk of thyroid crisis with this. These are tertiary care problems/questions. It is strongly advised that all babies born to women with thyroid disorder be under careful paediatric surveillance during their first two weeks of extra-uterine life.

Postpartum thyroid dysfunction

Postpartum thyroid dysfunction is far more common than is generally realised. Its incidence is quoted between 4–17% of pregnancies and is a separate entity from the pre-pregnancy and gestational onset thyroid disorders mentioned above. A mild thyrotoxic episode often develops 4–12 weeks postpartum, well after the formal postnatal examination. It presents with fatigue, depression and palpitations. Half will have a goitre and almost all will have anti-thyroid antibodies. Anti-thyroid drugs are rarely indicated although β-blockers may be useful. It usually resolves over the course of 2–3 months although around one third of women will go on to develop a hypothyroid state which can last for up to six months. A smaller number of women will apparently develop hypothyroidism without preceding hyperthyroidism. There is a strong association between postpartum thyroiditis and the development of thyroid disease in later life.

Thyrotoxic crisis

Thyrotoxic crisis is thankfully a rarity. It has a high maternal mortality rate. It presents with restlessness, tachycardia and fever, progressing to psychosis and coma. It may be precipitated by stress-related events, eg. infection or labour.

Tobacco

Tobacco is universally considered to be a toxin as far as pregnancy is concerned. Cotinine is detectable in the follicular fluid of women who smoke before ovulation. At the other end of pregnancy birth weights are lower and babies in smoking households are at a considerably enhanced risk of sudden infant death. The only pregnancy complication that appears to be reduced in smokers is pre-eclampsia. The wrong approach is to blackmail women who smoke in pregnancy. This produces guilt and may even cause an increase in tobacco consumption. Instead, a supportive and encouraging approach is recommended. A woman who cuts down on her smoking has done well even if she has failed to quit. Tobacco and smoking should be part of the preconceptual workup.

Vaccines

See *Table 7.14,* page 192. Vaccines may cause fetal infection and damage and are generally to be avoided in pregnancy. In some instances their use may be justified, for example, if there is a serious risk that withholding the vaccination could lead to greater harm (eg. poliomyelitis vaccine, yellow fever vaccine). The use of other vaccines may be indicated in certain circumstances (eg. tetanus toxoid, varicella-zoster immune globulin, hepatitis B vaccine). Data on anti-malarial prophylaxis is given in *Table 7.8.*

References

Bazire S (1998) *GP Psychotropic Handbook*. Quay Books, Dinton, Wiltshire

Briggs GG, Freeman RF, Yaffe SJ (1994) *Drugs in Pregnancy and Lactation,* 4 edn. Williams and Wilkins, New York

Jenner E (1996) *Immunisation Against Infectious Disease*. HMSO, London

Kassianos GC (1994) *Immunisation: Precautions and Contraindications,* 2 edn. Blackwells, Oxford

Further Reading

Drugs and Therapeutic Bulletin (1995) The practical management of thyroid disease in pregnancy. *Drug Therapeut Bull* **33**: 75–7

Ramsay I (1995) Thyroid disease. In: de Sweit M, ed. *Medical Disorders in Obstetric Practice,* 3 edn. Blackwells, Oxford

Table 7.14: Vaccines and immunoglobulins

Vaccine	Formulation	Notes
anthrax	alum antigen precipitate	no data
BCG	LIVE attenuated	although no problems noted, defer until puerperium if possible
botulism	antitoxin	
cholera	heat killed	not advised, only give if 'unavoidable'
diphtheria	formol toxoid	as DTP and DP. Avoid unless compelling risk
diphtheria	antitoxin	for passive immunisation
haemophylus B influenza	capsular polysaccharide	
hepatitis A	formaldehyde inactivated virus	not for use unless definite risk
hepatitis B	inactivated virus surface antigen	immunisation should not be withheld if woman is in high risk group
influenza	inactivated virus	give only if specific indication exists
measles	LIVE components as MR and MMR vaccine	AVOID PREGNANCY and 1 month (preferably 3) before pregnancy
meningococcal	polysaccharide	immunise if travelling to endemic area where benefit outweighs risk
mumps	LIVE attenuated as MMR	AVOID PREGNANCY
pertussis	killed organism	single agent and DTP. Avoid unless compelling risk
pneumococcal	polysaccharide	NOT for use in PREGNANCY
poliomyelitis	formol killed virus (Salk)	immunise if benefit appears to outweigh risk
rabies	freeze dried inactivated virus	pre-exposure vaccination only if risk is high
rubella	LIVE virus	AVOID PREGNANCY
smallpox	LIVE vaccinia	virtually no indication for use
tetanus	formol toxoid	
tuberculin	heat treated products	
typhoid	killed organisms	as with other vaccines, should only be given if clear indication exists
typhoid	Vi capsular polysaccharide	as with other vaccines, should only be given if clear indication exists
typhoid	LIVE attenuated	as with other vaccines, should only be given if clear indication exists
yellow fever	LIVE attenuated	immunise if travelling to endemic area where benefit outweighs risk
tick borne encephalitis	killed vaccine named patient basis	may be given in pregnancy if indicated (Kassianos, 1994)
Japanese B encephalitis	formol inactivated vaccine named patient basis	contraindicated in pregnancy
immunoglobulins	normal: gamma globulin etc	use only in specific risk situations, eg. rubella
	specific: tetanus, rabies, hepatitis B, varicella-zoster	use only in specific risk situations, eg. VZIG for chickenpox

Source: *Immunisation: Precautions and Contraindication; Immunisation Against Infectious Disease*

Notes:
* OPV should not be given to women during the first four months of pregnancy unless there are compelling reasons, eg. foreign travel

breast disorders

Data in this chapter is collected under two headings and aims to cover most primary care presentations of breast disorder. Breast cancer, although of paramount importance, is only briefly discussed as its diagnosis is generally made in the secondary care setting.

Chapter contents

Breast disorders in non-pregnant women

pain

lumps and nodularity

nipple discharge

breast infection

areolar and nipple disorder

pre-malignant conditions

duct ectasia

peri-ductal mastitis

breast cancer

mammography

silicone breast implants

other conditions

Breast disorders in pregnancy and the puerperium

antenatal preparation for lactation

breast carcinoma and lactation

breast pumps

contraception and lactation

engorgement

the HebsAg positive woman and lactation

the HIV positive woman and lactation

insufficient milk

mammoplasty and lactation

mastitis

nipple care

silicone implants and lactation

suppression of lactation

references

Table

Table 8.1: The pre-malignant potential of various breast disorders

Breast disorders in non-pregnant women

Disorders are listed below under symptoms and presentations rather than as disease entities. Breast cancer therefore is mentioned here under 'lumps and nodularity' and 'nipple discharge'. A very helpful table of suggestions and management for various breast problems can be found in *MIMS*. I keep a copy with this book for reference.

Pain

More commonly called mastalgia or mastodynia, breast pain is very common. Pain is a presenting feature in around 5% of cancers, but far more commonly it is a benign though not necessarily trivial problem. Severe mastalgia can interfere with the ability to work and normal family life and even place severe strains on relationships because of extreme tenderness. There are several common causes. Two-thirds of cases are cyclical in nature.

Cyclical mastalgia

Cyclical mastalgia is the commonest cause of significant breast discomfort. It usually peaks in the week prior to menstruation and typically affects the upper outer quadrants. Nodularity, which may also be cyclical, is common. It principally affects women in their twenties and thirties. It is usually considered as significant if it interferes with daily living activities. The following treatments are suggested:

- *reassurance* after thorough examination that the symptom is not the herald of sinister disease, supplemented with analgesic; may be all that is required
- *brassieres* should be well fitted and perhaps worn at night
- *caffeine reduction* helps some women, but only if initial consumption is high
- *dietary measures* which may help some women include reducing the amount of fat, especially saturated fats, and replacing the calories with carbohydrate
- *evening primrose oil* (capsules gamolenic acid 40 mg, 6–8/day) is safe and may be very effective if the symptoms are more severe. A response may take from four to six months to develop
- *danazol* is extremely effective. Usual starting dose is 200–300 mg/day which can be reduced to 100 mg/daily on alternate days after a month on the higher dose. Side-effects are not uncommon, but dose-dependent. It is teratogenic so contraception must be reliable
- *the combined oral contraceptive pill* will reduce or abolish symptoms in many women. Paradoxically it may cause mastalgia in a few women. Changing pill formulation or oestrogen dose may help. It is rarely used by secondary care specialists
- *bromocriptine* is reserved for specialist use. It is less effective than danazol but has a lower incidence of side-effects
- *HRT* may cause mastalgia which may be intolerable
- *ineffective remedies* include progestogens for the treatment of non-existent luteal phase defects, pyridoxine (vitamin B6: toxic effects of pyridoxine can be seen in prolonged treatment with doses of as little as 50 mg/day, although neurological problems are unusual with doses less than 200 mg/day for up to six months), antibiotics and diuretics for 'fluid

retention'. It must be remembered that the label 'ineffective' suggests that they are no better than placebos

- **placebo** will always have some effect in therapy especially in disorders which are essentially subjective. Always choose a safe placebo
- **in severe unresponsive cases** tamoxifen and GnRH analogues may be used. Usually initiated by secondary care professionals.

Non-cyclical mastalgia

Non-cyclical mastalgia is more commonly seen in women in their forties. It usually affects the inner quadrants and sub areolar areas of the breast. Nodularity is less common than in cyclic mastalgia. The presence of trigger spots is not unusual and these are occasionally amenable to surgical excision, although trigger spots may in fact be signs of underlying costochondritis. Histological analysis rarely detects the cause. Well fitting brassieres and the use of sleep/night brassieres are recommended. Endocrine treatments, evening primrose oil, bromocriptine and non-steroidal anti-inflammatories can be tried but their success rate is less than in cyclic mastalgia. NSAIDs are very useful for costochondritis. If trigger spots are identified, injection of local anaesthetic and steroids may be helpful (2 ml of 1% lignocaine and 40 mg/ml methylprednisolone). Excision of trigger spots is not infrequently followed by pain from the operation site and so is rarely performed.

Cancer

Cancer is an uncommon cause of mastalgia. Suspicion should be aroused if a new constant, consistent and unilateral breast pain develops. Pain and a mass requires urgent investigation.

Other causes

Other causes or differential diagnoses include Teite's syndrome (costochondritis) which is very common. Trauma, pregnancy, hyperprolactinaemia, cervical, thoracic vertebral disorder, thoracic outlet syndromes, lung and pleural conditions, and cholelithiasis are all rare causes.

Lumps and nodularity

Lumps and nodularity are common primary care presentations.

Normality

Normality is top of the list in the differential diagnosis. Some women are subject to recurrent and indistinct nodularity and lumpiness. If sinister disorder is excluded it should be labelled as 'benign breast disorder/change'.

Fibroadenoma

Fibroadenoma are a common benign, usually single, smooth mobile mass in younger women. They can, however, be multiple and recurrent. The giant fibroadenoma of adolescence is a variant.

Cyclical nodularity

Cyclical nodularity, previously called fibroadenosis and chronic cyclical mastitis. A benign breast disorder.

Cysts and pseudocysts (including galactocele)

Most breast cancer experts are firmly against generalists aspirating cysts. Cysts account for around 15% of all breast masses referred for a secondary care opinion. Multiple and recurrent cyst formation is associated with a marginally raised risk of breast cancer.

Cancer

Cancer is always the diagnosis to be excluded. The particular physical signs of importance are tethering to skin or deep structures, retraction of the nipple and a mass which is hard, irregular and immobile. The variations on the theme of breast cancer are numerous and a high index of suspicion must be maintained. Referral for a secondary care opinion should be prompt once the possibility of this diagnosis is entertained. Peri-menopausal and postmenopausal women should be referred for specialist opinion for any breast lumps. (See table in *MIMS* for specific advice).

Nipple discharge

This is not generally a sign of sinister disease although it usually evokes great anxiety in the patient, especially if it is bloody. It is usual to opt for mammography in women over 35 years of age with a nipple discharge.

Milky discharge

- **physiological**: related to pregnancy and the puerperium
- **drugs**: eg. phenothiazines, metoclopramide, oestrogens, opiates, methyldopa, Depo-Provera can cause galactorrhoea
- **pathological**: prolactinoma needs exclusion (check serum prolactin level, lateral skull X-rays are not the way to diagnose pituitary prolactinomas), ectopic prolactin secretion, hypothyroidism, renal failure

Coloured discharges

These range from creamy-coloured through green to black. They are not associated with an increased risk of cancer. Most are the consequence of duct ectasia (see below).

Bloody serous and watery discharges

Bloody serous and watery discharges are usually considered together. They require specialist investigation. The causes are:
- **duct papillomas** which are almost always benign
- **duct ectasia** see below
- **duct carcinomas** either invasive or *in situ*.

Breast infection

Breast infection can occur in the neonate as well as the adult breast. Neonatal mastitis is not discussed here. Lactational sepsis is discussed below.

Non-lactating breast infection

This presents either as central or peripheral infection:

- ***central and peri-areolar infection*** is usually the result of duct ectasia. The commonest infective organisms isolated are Staph' aureus, enterococci, bacterioides sp., and anaerobic streptococci. Antibiotics should be given early. Referral of resistant or repeated cases is recommended
- ***peripheral breast infections*** are less common. Older women and those with other disorders eg. diabetes mellitus, rheumatoid arthritis are more susceptible.

Skin sepsis

Skin sepsis on the breast tends to be seen in older women and especially in the obese. There is a link between sepsis and hygiene (or lack of it). Staph' aureus is the commonest isolate. Fungal infection may also occur. Flexural intertrigo often supports a cocktail of pathogens and opportunists. Attention to hygiene and choice of clothing is important in preventing recurrence. Tuberculosis of the breast is now a great rarity.

Factitious disease

Factitious disease should be kept as a differential diagnosis in odd, persistent or repetitive infections.

Areolar and nipple disorder

Inversion and retraction

Inversion may be a primary phenomenon where eversion has failed to occur. Secondary inversion or retraction of the nipple may be a sign of underlying breast cancer. Equally it may be caused by benign duct ectasia.

Eczema

Eczema can affect the nipple. Contact sensitises may be triggers. The principle differential is Paget's disease.

Montgomery's tubercles and sebaceous cysts

The areola has apocrine, modified sebaceous and rudimentary mammary glands, all of which can produce retention cysts. The tubercles described by Montgomery relate to the sebaceous gland hypertrophy sometimes seen in early pregnancy.

Trauma

Trauma, eg. joggers nipple due to friction.

Paget's disease of the nipple

Described by James Paget in 1874, this nipple disorder is a variety of breast carcinoma. It presents as a crusty, itchy eruption of the nipple prone to bleeding often without an obvious underlying breast mass. It accounts for 2% of breast cancers and peaks in incidence slightly later than other breast cancers at the age of 54.5 years. Confusion with eczema and dermatitis of the nipple are diagnostic pitfalls. Three stages may be identified:

- **itching and/or burning** of a normal or slightly reddened and perhaps smooth nipple
- **crusting of the nipple**. There may be associated discharge onto garments. This may progress to erosion and crevicing of the nipple
- **erosion of entire nipple** spreading at first to the areola which contracts and then to the skin of the breast itself.

Rarities

Rarities include leiomyoma of the muscular fibres of the areola and nipple, erosive adenomatosis which produces recurrent painful ulcers, crusts and induration. Raynaud's phenomena can affect the nipple.

Pre-malignant conditions

Table 8.1: The pre-malignant potential of various breast disorders

No increased risk	Slight increased risk 1.5–2x	Moderate increased risk >2x
fibroadenoma, adenoma, cysts, duct ectasia, inflammatory mastitis, periductal mastitis, squamous metaplasia	hyperplasia, papillomas with fibroepithelial core	atypical hyperplasia of duct or lobule, lobular carcinoma in situ, ductal carcinoma in situ

Source: *Benign Disorders and Diseases of the Breast* (1989), Hughes *et al*

Hyperplasia is associated with a marginally raised risk of breast cancer in women with a first degree relative who already has breast cancer

Duct ectasia

Ectasia or dilation of ducts is commonly seen as a part of the involutional process which begins to affect the breast from about the age of thirty. It rarely presents until later life. It is present in just under half of all 70-year-old women. The process presents as a spectrum of changes ranging from the physiological to the pathological. In its more florid form it has parallels with bronchiectasis and sialectasis. Ducts, which are generally 1 mm or less in diameter, dilate to up to 5 mm.

- **secretions** may cause a nipple discharge. It may be sero-sanguinous, watery or coloured, but not milky
- **peri-ductal inflammation** may result from stagnation of secretions
- **infection** may supervene and lead to sub-areolar abscess and duct fistulae
- **mastalgia** may result from this inflammation
- **nipple retraction** may result from scarring and fibrosis. Typically, it slowly buries the nipple under a slit-like opening in the areola in older women

Peri-ductal mastitis

Peri-ductal mastitis is a distinct condition which is related to duct ectasia. It typically produces an area of central or peri-areolar mastitis in women who are in their thirties and who smoke. Initial treatment is with antibiotics. Abscess, nipple retraction and fistula formation are complications. Recurrent or persistent disorder should be treated by excision of the diseased duct.

Breast cancer

It is not appropriate to provide a detailed discussion of breast cancer here as it is mainly a secondary care problem.

- ***oral contraception and breast cancer***: the Collaborative Group on Hormonal Contraception and Breast Cancer, 1996 reported a higher incidence of breast cancer in users of oral contraceptives. The rise was slight, waned on cessation of treatment and was gone by ten years. The excess cancers were few in number but more likely to be localised to the breast than in 'never users' of the pill.

Mammography

Mammography can be offered as a screening tool or as a diagnostic investigation because of clinical indication. There is also a place for mammography in selected premenopausal women, particularly those with a significant family history of breast cancer (at least one first degree relative with the disease) and also in women with very large breasts. It is known that manual examination is difficult in women with very large and fatty breasts and that mammography is more sensitive. In young women, the prevalence of breast cancer is so low that mammography cannot be justified. There is, however, argument about the age where the risk/benefit ratio of mammography screening changes. It is probably somewhere in the mid to late forties. There is also argument about the frequency of screening. Individuals may benefit from yearly screening but communities benefit from screening two or three-yearly (see 'General principles' under 'Screening in Gynaecology, *Chapter 1*). Two-view mammography is superior to one-view (Margolese, 1996). Women over 35 years with symptomatic breast disease or a lump should be considered for mammography.

Silicone breast implants

Concerns that silicone breast implants can cause rheumatic conditions have been voiced for some years. This led to the American FDA banning their use pending more data in 1992. The situation in the UK is different with the Chief Medical Officer stating that there was insufficient evidence to show a risk of developing rheumatoid arthritis, SLE, etc. A recent study from the United States found a significant but small increase in incidence of rheumatic disorder among women who had silicone implants compared with women who did not (Hennekens, 1996). The study was susceptible to reporting bias and, although it is possible that there is no heightened risk, at worst the risk appears slight. Despite the lack of evidence that silicone breast implants are causatively related to the development of connective tissue disease the FDA has maintained a moratorium on their use for several years. A recent Swedish study comparing women who had implants for cosmetic or post cancer reconstructive purposes with matched women following breast reduction surgery found no link between breast implants and connective tissue disease (Nyren O, 1998). The recent NHS messaging service cascade (March, 1999) relates not to silicone breast implants but rather to soya oil filled implants. The Medical Devices Agency has recommended no more soya oil filled implants be fitted until concerns about long term safety are clarified. These implants are also known as Trilucent Breast Implants.

Other conditions

Other conditions include fat necrosis following trauma which can mimic carcinoma. A fatty pseudo-cyst may develop which can be aspirated (refer such cases to secondary care); lipomas are not uncommon in the breast; and parfinomas may be seen occasionally in older women who had paraffin injections in the past as a form of augmentation mammoplasty. Refer all of these cases on to a specialist.

Breast disorders in pregnancy and the puerperium

● **Antenatal preparation for lactation**

Antenatal preparation for lactation falls into two categories. Firstly, it is thought that positive encouragement and advice about breast feeding at antenatal classes increases the numbers of women who go on to breast feed. Secondly, nipple preparation or 'conditioning' to 'toughen up' for the mechanical traumas of suckling has not been shown to be effective (Enkin *et al*, 1989).

● **Breast carcinoma and lactation**

Previous breast carcinoma is not commonly encountered in the lactation period. Previous surgery may have damaged ducts but more importantly radiotherapy may have irreversibly damaged glandular tissue. The consequence in these women is that unilateral lactation failure is likely, although if breast feeding is desired by the mother she can be reassured that it is as likely to be successful from the other breast. Few studies have addressed the effect of lactation on long term prognosis but what evidence there is suggests, if anything, that it is slightly beneficial.

● Breast pumps

Plastic hand pumps can be prescribed on an FP10. Electric pumps can be hired, usually through the local National Childbirth Trust group.

● Contraception and lactation

The oestrogen component of the combined oral contraceptive pill appears to reduce milk volume. Although many women use combined pills and lactate successfully the incidence of lactation failure and early supplementary feeding is significantly higher. In developing countries this can be disastrous. In the UK the risks of lactation failure have to be weighed against the benefits of reliable contraception case by case. The progestogen only pill does not appear to interfere with lactation. Pills containing levonorgestrel should be avoided as significant amounts of this hormone transfer to the milk.

● Engorgement

This occurs when milk production is in excess of that taken by the baby. In cases where lactation is continuing attention to correct positioning and latching on is vital. This is because milk remains or continues to flow into the ducts under the areola after feeding. The result is back pressure, pain and if pressure forces milk through the walls of ducts into the tissues, sterile mastitis. The treatments are the encouragement of unrestricted access of the baby for feeding and if mastitis has developed, manual expression of the breast. The critical importance of correct positioning of the baby on the breast is to be stressed.

● The HepBsAg positive woman and lactation

Lactation in the HepBsAg positive woman is to be encouraged as long as immunoprophylaxis of the infant has been started (see *Chapter 6* and Gupta, 1997).

● The HIV positive woman and lactation

Lactation in the HIV positive woman is to be discouraged in countries like the UK where safe formula milks are available. Transmission of virus occurs around the time of delivery. Caesarean section reduces the risk of transmission. In those infants not infected, exposure to breast milk poses a definite hazard.

NB: This is not the same as having HIV antibodies (babies have these passively from their HIV positive mothers for some months after birth).

● Insufficient milk

Insufficient milk is thought to occur in less than 5% of women. The most common cause appears to be prevention of unrestricted access of the baby to the breast. Test weighing before and after feeding is a very poor guide to milk output and is not recommended. In cases of true insufficient milk production, where the baby's weight gain is inadequate, supplementation is advisable. Studies on the use of oxytocin and dopaminergic drugs are underway but cannot at this stage be recommended.

● Mammoplasty and lactation

Previous mammoplasty and lactation is performed frequently in young women. In some cases breast size is augmented and in others reduced. A recent review of cases of augmentation mammoplasty from the United States found lactation insufficiency in 64% compared with just 7% among controls who had not had breast surgery. The majority of women in this study had undergone surgery for cosmetic reasons. The particular surgical approach was found to be important. In addition to reducing nipple sensation, peri-areolar incisions are likely to cut lactiferous ducts which drain radially onto the nipple. Submammary and axilliary approaches interfere less.

● Mastitis

Mastitis can be sterile as a result of engorgement and extravasation of milk into the breast tissue or infective. Sterile mastitis and engorgement can be complicated by infection. Bacteria can also enter the breast through cracks and abrasions in the nipple. Infective mastitis will present with systemic symptoms and signs in addition to those of local inflammation. Infective mastitis needs urgent and vigorous treatment with broad spectrum antibiotics.

● Nipple care

Nipple care (see also antenatal preparation for lactation). The importance of correct positioning of the baby on the breast cannot be stressed too highly. Poor latching on with the baby sucking the nipple rather that milking the whole areola and pulling in its surrounding skin is the source of sore and cracked nipples. This causes pain, interferes with happy bonding and can lead to mastitis and breast abscess. The critical factor is to ensure that the baby's lower lip and gum oppose the skin below the areola and that plenty of breast enters the mouth. The nipple should not be sucked or chewed at all. A skilled breast feeding adviser is crucial. Nipple shields can be used but are generally disliked by both mothers and babies and may lead to insufficient milk production if used more than briefly.

● Silicone implants and lactation

The data is inconclusive. One study in the USA suggested that oesophageal disorders resembling those seen in scleroderma may occur more commonly among babies breast fed by silicone breast augmented mothers. Correspondence in the journals subsequently cast doubt on the conclusions of the study. An association has not been proved but a relationship may exist (Epstein 1996, Levine 1996).

● Suppression of lactation

This is traditionally achieved by avoiding any nipple stimulation from the baby, wearing a firm supporting brassiere day and night supplemented with analgesics if required. The use of high doses of oestrogen to suppress lactation has been abandoned because of the significant danger of venous thrombosis. Bromocriptine can be given. The dose is 2.5 mg per day for two or three days rising to 2.5 mg twice daily for a further fourteen days. It is contraindicated in hypertensive women and those with coronary artery disease or serious mental disorder. Blood pressure should be monitored during treatment. Milk production may return when the course is finished. Bromocriptine is usually reserved for use in mothers after perinatal death, but in view of its potential for significant side-effects there is an argument for avoiding its use unless lactation suppression is vital and the mother makes an informed decision to use it.

References

The Collaborative Group on Hormonal Contraception and Breast Cancer (1996) Breast Cancer and hormonal contraceptives: collaborative re-analysis of individual data on 53,297 women with breast cancer and 100,239 women without breast cancer from 54 epidemiological studies. *Lancet* **347**: 1713–27

Enkin M, Keirse M, Chalmers I (1989) *A Guide to Effective Care in Pregnancy and Childbirth*. Oxford University Press, Oxford

Epstein WA (1996) Silicone breast implants and scleroderma like oesophageal disease in breast fed infants. *JAMA* **275**: 184–5

Gupta S *et al* (1997) Women and HIV. *Br J Fam Plan*, **23**: 83–7

Hennekens CH *et al*, (1996) Self reported breast implants and connective-tissue diseases in female health professionals. *JAMA* **275**: 616–21

Hughes LE, Mansel RE, Webster DJT (1989) *Benign Disorders and Diseases of the Breast*. Ballière Tindall, London

Levine JJ (1996) Silicone breast implants and scleroderma like oesophageal disease in breast fed infants. *JAMA* **275**: 185

Margolese R (1996) Screening mammography in young women: a different perspective. *Lancet* **347**: 881–2

Nyren O *et al* (1998) Risk of connective tissue disease and related disorders among women with breast implants: a nationwide retrospective study in Sweden. *Br Med J* **316**: 417–22

Index